Contents

Chapter 1: Introduction to Feng Shui

In the tapestry of ancient Chinese philosophy, Feng Shui emerges as a vibrant thread, weaving through the ages to guide us in the harmonious dance between energy and our living spaces. As we embark on this journey of discovery, let us unfurl the pages of history to understand the genesis of Feng Shui and the profound impact it continues to exert on our lives.

The Origins of Feng Shui

Feng Shui, pronounced "fung shway," translates to "wind-water" in English. Its roots trace back over 3,000 years to ancient China, where it evolved as a complex system intertwining Taoist and Confucian principles. The early practitioners of Feng Shui observed the natural world, seeking to comprehend the subtle forces that governed the universe. They discovered that the alignment of physical spaces could influence the flow of Qi, the vital life force that animates all living things.

Philosophical Foundations of Feng Shui

At its core, Feng Shui is deeply embedded in the philosophical traditions of Yin and Yang and the Five Elements. The concept of Yin and Yang symbolizes the duality inherent in nature—dark and light, feminine and masculine, receptive and active. Understanding and balancing these opposing forces lie at the heart of Feng Shui, aiming to create equilibrium in our surroundings.

The Five Elements—Wood, Fire, Earth, Metal, and Water—form another crucial pillar of Feng Shui philosophy. These elements are not merely physical substances but represent dynamic energies that interact with one another. By harnessing and harmonizing these elements, practitioners seek to optimize the flow of Qi, promoting health, prosperity, and overall well-being.

The Three Schools of Feng Shui

Over time, three distinct schools of Feng Shui emerged, each with its unique approach to harmonizing energy. The Form School emphasizes the physical features of the environment, advocating for the strategic placement of mountains, rivers, and structures. The Compass School, on the other hand, relies on the use of a compass to determine the direction and alignment of spaces, while the Black Hat Sect Feng Shui incorporates spiritual and intuitive elements into its practice.

Feng Shui in Everyday Life

Feng Shui is not an esoteric concept reserved for scholars and sages; it is a practical and accessible art that anyone can integrate into their daily lives. At its essence, Feng Shui invites us to become co-creators of our environments, shaping spaces that resonate with positive energy and foster harmony.

As we navigate the chapters ahead, we will uncover the secrets of the Bagua Map, explore the balance of Yin and Yang, and delve into specific applications for health, wealth, relationships, and more. By understanding and applying the principles of Feng Shui, we embark on a transformative journey—one where our living spaces become not only shelters but sanctuaries that nurture and empower every facet of our lives. So, let us embark on this exploration, guided by the ancient wisdom of Feng Shui, as we learn to dance with the wind and flow with the water, harmonizing the energies that surround us.

Chapter 2: The Five Elements in Feng Shui

In the intricate tapestry of Feng Shui, the Five Elements stand as vibrant hues, each contributing its unique energy to the canvas of our living spaces. As we unravel the essence of these elements—Wood, Fire, Earth, Metal, and Water—we embark on a journey to understand how their dynamic interplay shapes the flow of Qi and, consequently, our well-being.

Wood: The Essence of Growth and Vitality

In the realm of Feng Shui, Wood embodies the energy of growth, expansion, and vitality. Picture a flourishing tree, its branches reaching towards the sky—the epitome of Wood energy. This element is associated with new beginnings, creativity, and the spring season. To infuse your living spaces with Wood energy, consider incorporating wooden furniture, lush plants, and vibrant green hues. By nurturing the Wood element, you foster a sense of renewal and continuous evolution in your surroundings.

Fire: Igniting Passion and Transformation

Fire, with its radiant warmth and transformative power, represents the essence of passion and change in Feng Shui. Picture a crackling fireplace or the vibrant hues of a sunset—this is the energy of Fire. Introduce candles, bold colours like red and orange, and triangular shapes to infuse your spaces with the dynamic spirit of Fire. Balancing Fire energy can ignite inspiration, foster courage, and kindle the flames of positive transformation in your life.

Earth: Grounding Stability ad Nourishment

At the core of stability and nourishment lies the Earth element in Feng Shui. Picture the solid ground beneath your feet, the rich soil that sustains life. Earth energy promotes grounding, stability, and a sense of security. Introduce earthy colours, square shapes, and ceramic or terracotta elements to enhance the Earth energy in your spaces. By anchoring yourself in the nurturing embrace of Earth, you cultivate a foundation for balance and harmony in your home and life.

Metal: The Essence of Precision and Clarity

Metal, with its precision and clarity, embodies the qualities of organization and focus on Feng Shui. Imagine the gleam of polished metal surfaces or the crispness of autumn air—this is the energy of Metal. Integrate metal decor, white and metallic colours, and circular shapes to invite the purifying essence of Metal into your spaces. By doing so, you promote mental clarity, organization, and a sense of precision, fostering an environment conducive to productivity and efficiency.

Water: The Fluid Essence of Adaptability

Flowing like a tranquil river or crashing like powerful waves, Water represents adaptability and the ability to overcome obstacles in Feng Shui. Picture the soothing sound of raindrops or the reflective surface of a pond. To harness Water energy, incorporate flowing water features, mirrors, and deep, dark colours into your spaces. By embracing the fluidity of Water, you encourage adaptability, intuition, and the removal of stagnant energy in your surroundings.

The Dance of the Elements in Harmony

The magic of Feng Shui lies in the harmonious dance of these Five Elements. To optimize the flow of Qi in your spaces, seek a balanced representation of all elements. The absence or dominance of any particular element can disrupt the equilibrium, affecting the energy dynamics within your home or workplace.

As we move forward in our exploration of Feng Shui, remember that the art lies not just in recognizing the individual elements but in orchestrating their dance—creating a symphony of energy that resonates with the rhythm of your life. In the upcoming chapters, we'll delve deeper into the application of these elements in specific areas of your home and life, unlocking the secrets to a harmonious and balanced existence.

Chapter 3: The Bagua Map: Blueprint for Harmonious Living

In the profound tapestry of Feng Shui, the Bagua Map emerges as a sacred blueprint—a guide to aligning our spaces with the natural forces that govern the universe. Rooted in ancient Chinese philosophy, the Bagua Map is a powerful tool that enables us to map out different areas of our homes and lives, facilitating the optimization of energy flow and fostering harmony in every aspect. As we step into the intricate world of the Bagua Map, we embark on a transformative journey, discovering the keys to unlocking the full potential of our living spaces.

Understanding the Bagua Map

At its essence, the Bagua Map is an octagonal grid, each side representing a specific aspect of life. Derived from the I Ching, an ancient Chinese divination text, the Bagua organizes these aspects into eight guas, each associated with a particular element, colour, and life area. These guas are Wealth, Fame, Love and Marriage, Family, Health, Creativity, Wisdom, and Career.

Activating the Bagua Map

To activate the Bagua Map in your home, align it with the main entrance, ensuring that the guas correspond with the various rooms and areas. Imagine the Bagua as a transparent overlay, laid upon your floor plan, with the bottom of the octagon facing the entrance. This alignment allows you to identify specific life areas within your living spaces, providing a roadmap for enhancing energy flow and creating a harmonious environment.

The Eight Guas of the Bagua Map

Wealth (Xun Gua):

Associated with the element Wood and the colour green, the Wealth gua pertains to abundance and prosperity. To activate this area, consider incorporating plants, wooden elements, and symbols of wealth such as coins or wealth bowls.

Fame and Reputation (Li Gua):

Aligned with the element Fire and the colour red, the Fame gua is linked to recognition and reputation. Enhance this area with fiery decor, bold colours, and symbols that represent your personal achievements and aspirations.

Love and Marriage (Kun Gua):

Represented by the element Earth and the colour pink or red, the Love and Marriage gua focuses on relationships. Strengthen this area with romantic decor, pairs of items, and imagery that symbolizes love and commitment.

Family (Zhen Gua):

Aligned with the element Wood and the colour green, the Family gua centres around unity and connection. Infuse this space with images of family, plants, and elements that evoke a sense of growth and support.

Health (Tai Qi Gua):

Associated with the element Earth and the colour yellow, the Health gua emphasizes well-being and balance. Prioritize cleanliness, incorporate earthy tones, and introduce elements that promote a healthy and nurturing atmosphere.

Creativity and Children (Qian Gua):

Represented by the element Metal and the colour white, the Creativity gua encourages the flow of artistic energy and innovation. Nurture this area with artwork, creative tools, and symbols that inspire imagination.

Wisdom (Dui Gua):

Aligned with the element Metal and the colour white, the Wisdom gua focuses on knowledge and self-improvement. Foster this area with books, learning materials, and symbols that reflect your pursuit of wisdom and personal growth.

Career (Kan Gua):

Associated with the element Water and the colour black, the Career gua embodies your professional journey. Strengthen this area with water features, reflective surfaces, and symbols that represent your career goals and aspirations.

Activating the Bagua in Specific Areas

As you align the Bagua Map with your living spaces, consider the unique characteristics of each gua and the corresponding adjustments you can make to optimize the energy flow:

Main Entrance:

The main entrance serves as the mouth of Qi, welcoming energy into your home. Ensure it is well-lit, clutter-free, and inviting to encourage positive energy to flow in.

Bedroom:

The bedroom is a sanctuary for rest and rejuvenation. Activate the appropriate gua to enhance specific aspects of your life, such as love and relationships in the Love and Marriage gua.

Kitchen:

The heart of nourishment, the kitchen is linked to the Health gua. Keep it clean, organized, and filled with fresh, wholesome ingredients to promote well-being.

Home Office:

Activate the Career gua in your home office to boost professional growth and success. Introduce water features, inspirational decor, and symbols of achievement.

Living Room:

Infuse the living room with elements that correspond to the desired guas, creating a balanced and harmonious space for socializing, relaxation, and creativity.

Bathroom:

Bathrooms are associated with the Water element. Keep them well-maintained and introduce elements that promote a sense of cleanliness and purification.

The Power of Intention and Symbolism

Beyond the physical adjustments, the Bagua Map encourages us to imbue our spaces with intention and symbolism. Consider incorporating personal items, images, and symbols that hold significant meaning to you. This infusion of personal energy adds a layer of authenticity, aligning your living spaces with your aspirations and desires.

The Reflective Nature of the Bagua Map

As you navigate the intricate energy map of the Bagua, remember that it is not a static guide but a reflection of the dynamic nature of life. Changes in circumstances, goals, and personal growth may warrant adjustments to the Bagua activations in your living spaces. Regularly reassess and realign the Bagua Map to ensure that it continues to resonate with the evolving energy of your life.

The Bagua Map, with its octagonal wisdom, offers a profound framework for harmonizing our living spaces with the universal energies that surround us. As we explore the intricacies of each gua and align our environments with intention and purpose, we unlock the potential for transformative change in every facet of our lives.

In the chapters ahead, we will delve deeper into specific applications of the Bagua Map, exploring advanced techniques, case studies, and real-life examples that highlight the profound impact of aligning our spaces with the sacred geometry of Feng Shui. So, with the Bagua Map as our guide, let us continue this enlightening journey, unlocking the secrets to a harmonious and balanced existence.

Chapter 4: Yin and Yang in Feng Shui: Balancing Dualities for Harmonious Living

In the rich tapestry of Feng Shui, the ancient Chinese philosophy of Yin and Yang stands as a profound guide to understanding the dualities that shape our existence. Yin and Yang represent the dynamic interplay of opposites—dark and light, feminine and masculine, receptive and active. As we delve into the depths of Chapter 4, we uncover the philosophical foundations of Yin and Yang, exploring how these complementary forces influence the flow of energy in our living spaces and illuminate the path to harmony.

The Essence of Yin and Yang

Yin and Yang are fundamental concepts deeply rooted in Chinese cosmology and Taoist philosophy. They symbolize the eternal dance of opposites, where each force contains the seed of its counterpart. Yin is associated with qualities such as receptivity, passivity, darkness, and the feminine, while Yang embodies activity, brightness, masculinity, and assertiveness. Together, they form a harmonious whole, with each containing a trace of the other.

The Tai Chi Symbol: Unity in Duality

The Tai Chi symbol, often recognized as the Yin-Yang symbol, visually encapsulates the essence of this philosophy. In this circular emblem, a white and a black segment swirl together in a perpetual dance. Within the white segment, there is a black dot, and vice versa, symbolizing the inherent presence of each force within the other. This symbol reflects the cyclical nature of life, where one force transforms into the other, creating a continuous, balanced flow.

Yin and Yang in Nature

Observing nature provides profound insights into the principles of Yin and Yang. Consider the cycle of day and night—Yang's brilliance yielding to Yin's tranquility as the sun sets. The changing seasons also embody this dance, with the vibrant growth of spring (Yang) giving way to the introspective rest of winter (Yin). Understanding and aligning with these natural cycles allow us to harness the inherent energy of Yin and Yang in our living spaces.

Application of Yin and Yang in Feng Shui

In Feng Shui, the balance of Yin and Yang is pivotal for optimizing the flow of Qi—the vital life force that animates our environments. Creating harmony involves recognizing the predominant energies in each space and making intentional adjustments to strike a balance. Here's how Yin and Yang principles manifest in different areas of our homes:

Living Room:

In the living room, balance the active energy of socializing and entertainment (Yang) with elements that promote relaxation and tranquility (Yin). Incorporate comfortable furniture, soft textures, and subdued lighting to create a harmonious blend.

Bedroom:

The bedroom, a sanctuary for rest, benefits from a Yin-dominant atmosphere. Soft bedding, dim lighting, and soothing colours contribute to a restful environment, supporting rejuvenating sleep and balanced energy.

Kitchen:

The kitchen, often a hub of activity and culinary creativity (Yang), benefits from introducing Yin elements to balance the energy. Consider incorporating calming colours, comfortable seating, and elements that promote a sense of nourishment and harmony.

Home Office:

Balancing the dynamic energy of work (Yang) with elements that foster focus and tranquility (Yin) is crucial in a home office. Introduce natural light, plants, and organization to create a space conducive to both productivity and mental well-being.

Bathroom:

Bathrooms, associated with the Water element and a Yin quality, benefit from balancing the stillness of water with vibrant, uplifting elements. Consider introducing plants, bright colours, and natural scents to infuse the space with positive energy.

Yin and Yang in Furniture and Decor

Feng Shui extends its influence on the choice of furniture and decor within our spaces. Understanding the inherent qualities of Yin and Yang aids in making intentional selections:

Furniture:

Choose furniture that balances the energies of Yin and Yang. Soft, rounded shapes and plush fabrics contribute Yin qualities, while angular, sturdy furniture leans towards Yang. Striking a balance in the shapes and materials within a room creates visual harmony.

Colour Palette:

Colours play a pivotal role in expressing Yin and Yang energies. Cool, muted tones and pastels are Yin, while bold, warm colours lean towards Yang. Harmonizing these colour energies throughout your home creates a cohesive and balanced atmosphere.

Textures:

Soft textures, such as plush carpets and cosy blankets, contribute Yin qualities, while sleek, hard surfaces embody Yang. Introducing a variety of textures within a space creates a sensory balance that promotes overall harmony.

Balancing Yin and Yang in Specific Life Areas

Applying Yin and Yang principles to specific life areas enhances the overall energy flow in your home:

Health and Well-being:

In spaces dedicated to health and well-being, create a balance between active exercise areas (Yang) and serene relaxation corners (Yin). Integrate natural elements, such as plants and calming colours, to promote holistic well-being.

Relationships:

Foster harmonious relationships by balancing shared activity spaces (Yang) with intimate, comfortable corners (Yin). Creating an environment that supports both connection and personal space enhances the dynamics of relationships.

Career and Success:

In your workspace, balance the active, focused energy of productivity (Yang) with elements that promote clarity and mental well-being (Yin). Natural light, organization, and calming decor contribute to a balanced and supportive career environment.

The Ever-Changing Dance of Yin and Yang

Recognizing that Yin and Yang are not fixed but ever-changing energies is crucial in the practice of Feng Shui. Seasons, life events, and personal growth all contribute to the dynamic interplay of these forces. Regular assessments and adjustments in alignment with the evolving energies allow for a continuous flow of harmonious Qi.

Case Studies: Balancing Yin and Yang in Living Spaces

To deepen our understanding of Yin and Yang in Feng Shui, let's explore a few case studies illustrating how intentional adjustments can transform the energy dynamics in different living spaces:

Case Study 1: Tranquil Bedroom Transformation

Challenge: A couple sought to create a serene and restful bedroom.

Solution: Introducing Yin elements such as soft lighting, calming colours, and plush bedding transformed the bedroom into a sanctuary, fostering deeper sleep and connection.

Case Study 2: Harmonizing Family Dynamics

Challenge: A busy family sought to create a harmonious living room.

Solution: Balancing the active energy of family gatherings (Yang) with comfortable seating, soft textures, and calming decor (Yin) created a space that supported both connection and individual relaxation.

Case Study 3: Productive Home Office

Challenge: A professional working from home wanted to enhance productivity.

Solution: Balancing the active energy of work with elements promoting focus and tranquility, such as natural light, plants, and organization, created an environment conducive to both productivity and well-being.

As we conclude our exploration of Yin and Yang in Feng Shui, we

recognize that the delicate dance of these dual forces forms the very fabric of harmonious living. By understanding and embracing the dynamic interplay of Yin and Yang in our living spaces, we unlock the potential to create environments that support balance, well-being, and positive energy flow.

In the chapters to come, we will delve even deeper into the practical applications of Yin and Yang, exploring advanced techniques, case studies, and real-life examples that highlight the transformative power of harmonizing these opposing forces. From intentional furniture arrangements to mindful decor choices, every aspect of our living spaces can be curated to honor the principles of Yin and Yang.

As we navigate the intricate landscape of Feng Shui, guided by the wisdom of ancient Chinese philosophy, let us embrace the ever-changing dance of Yin and Yang. By doing so, we not only enhance the energy dynamics within our homes but also cultivate a deeper connection with the fundamental forces that shape our lives. So, with a newfound understanding of Yin and Yang, let us continue our journey toward creating spaces that resonate with balance, harmony, and the vibrant energy of life.

Chapter 5: Feng Shui for Health and Wellness: Nurturing Harmony in Living Spaces

In the intricate philosophy of Feng Shui, the interconnectedness of our living environments and our well-being takes centre stage. Chapter 5 delves into the profound ways in which Feng Shui can be harnessed to cultivate and enhance health and wellness. By weaving together, the principles of energy flow, symbolism, and intentional design, Feng Shui offers a holistic approach to creating spaces that nurture physical, mental, and spiritual harmony.

The Holistic Perspective: Health in Mind, Body, and Spirit

Health, according to traditional Chinese philosophy, extends beyond the physical realm, encompassing the balance of mind, body, and spirit. Feng Shui recognizes this holistic perspective and views our living spaces as a canvas where the energies of these dimensions converge. By fostering positive energy, known as Qi, within our surroundings, we lay the foundation for a holistic approach to well-being.

Qi Flow and the Living Environment: A Foundation for Vitality

Central to Feng Shui is the concept of Qi flow—a dynamic, harmonious movement of energy within our living spaces. When Qi flows freely and unobstructed, it contributes to a vibrant and healthy environment. Understanding how to optimize Qi flow involves a deliberate arrangement of furniture, thoughtful use of colours, and a mindful selection of materials.

Clutter Clearance:

Clutter acts as a barrier to the smooth flow of Qi, creating stagnant energy pockets that can impact health negatively. The Bagua Map, introduced in Chapter 3, is a useful tool to identify areas associated with health. Decluttering and organizing these areas facilitate the circulation of fresh, positive energy, promoting a sense of order and vitality.

Air and Light Quality:

Essential to well-being is the quality of air and light within our living spaces. Proper ventilation, an abundance of natural light, and the introduction of indoor plants contribute to a healthy atmosphere. Adequate ventilation ensures the circulation of fresh air, while natural light has a profound impact on mood and overall vitality.

Furniture Arrangement:

The arrangement of furniture plays a pivotal role in Qi flow. Avoid blocking pathways and ensure that furniture layouts allow for easy movement. In the bedroom, for instance, position the bed to have a clear view of the room's entrance, promoting a sense of security and openness while optimizing energy circulation.

Colour Psychology:

Colours, with their psychological impact, play a significant role in influencing our well-being. Feng Shui assigns specific colours to each of the five elements, and choosing the right colours for different areas of your home contributes to a harmonious energy balance. For spaces associated with health, consider incorporating soothing colours like greens, blues, and earth tones.

Natural Materials:

Infusing natural materials into your living spaces aligns with the Earth element in Feng Shui and contributes to a grounded and healthy environment. Wood, stone, and fabrics made from natural fibres foster a connection with the natural world, promoting a sense of balance and well-being.

The Bedroom: A Sanctuary for Restful Sleep and Healing

In Feng Shui, the bedroom holds a special significance as a sanctuary for rest, rejuvenation, and healing. The intentional arrangement of elements within the bedroom contributes to a space that supports physical and mental well-being.

Bed Placement:

The bed, being the focal point of the bedroom, is crucial to consider in the context of Feng Shui. Position the bed in a commanding position, ensuring a clear view of the bedroom entrance while avoiding direct alignment with it. This arrangement enhances a sense of security, promoting a restful atmosphere conducive to healing and vitality.

Colour Choices:

Selecting calming and restful colours for the bedroom is essential. Soft blues, greens, or neutral tones create a tranquil ambiance, fostering relaxation and supporting quality sleep. Avoid overly stimulating colours that may disrupt the serene atmosphere necessary for optimal well-being.

Balancing Yin and Yang:

Striking a balance between Yin and Yang energies is crucial in the bedroom. Incorporate soft textures, gentle lighting, and soothing decor to enhance Yin qualities, while maintaining order and cleanliness contributes Yang qualities. This balance creates an environment that supports both restful sleep and wakeful rejuvenation.

Electronics and EMF Considerations:

Minimize the presence of electronic devices in the bedroom, as they emit electromagnetic fields (EMFs) that can interfere with sleep and overall health. Create a technology-free zone by keeping smartphones, tablets, and other electronic devices away from the sleeping area.

Symbolic Imagery:

Infuse the bedroom with symbols of health, love, and positivity. Artwork depicting serene landscapes, images of loved ones, or symbols associated with well-being can contribute to a positive and uplifting atmosphere, promoting overall health and balance.

The Kitchen: Nourishing the Body and Soul

The kitchen, often considered the heart of the home, plays a crucial role in fostering health and wellness. Applying Feng Shui principles to the kitchen involves mindful design choices and intentional practices that support vitality.

Cleanliness and Organization:

A clean and organized kitchen is essential for maintaining a positive energy flow. Regularly declutter countertops, clean appliances, and organize storage spaces to prevent the accumulation of stagnant energy. A well-maintained kitchen not only enhances efficiency but also contributes to a sense of well-being.

Stove Placement:

The stove is a focal point in Feng Shui, symbolizing wealth and well-being. Position the stove so that the cook has a clear view of the kitchen entrance, reflecting a sense of control and security. Keeping the stove in good working condition symbolizes the steady flow of nourishing energy and contributes to overall health.

Colours and Elements:

Integrate colours associated with nourishment and vitality in the kitchen. Shades of green and yellow are particularly auspicious. Incorporate elements of the Wood element, such as wooden utensils and cutting boards, to enhance the natural and vibrant energy of the kitchen.

Healthy Eating Environment:

Cultivate a space that encourages healthy eating habits. Create a dedicated area for eating, preferably away from the stove, to promote mindful and enjoyable meals. Ensure that the dining area is well-lit and inviting, contributing to a positive and health-conscious atmosphere.

Wellness Symbols:

Infuse the kitchen with symbols of health and abundance. Display fresh fruits, vegetables, and herbs prominently, and consider incorporating symbols or artwork that evoke a sense of vitality and well-being. These symbols serve as daily reminders to make health-conscious choices in the kitchen.

The Bathroom: A Sanctuary for Purification and Renewal

While the bathroom is associated with the Water element and is often seen as a space for cleansing, it can also contribute to overall well-being with mindful Feng Shui practices.

Ventilation and Lighting:

Adequate ventilation is essential in the bathroom to prevent stagnant energy. Ensure proper air circulation and maximize natural light when possible. Consider using full-spectrum lighting to mimic natural sunlight, contributing to a sense of purity and renewal.

Colour Choices:

Choose calming colours for the bathroom, such as soft blues, greens, or neutral tones. Avoid overly bright or stark colours, as they may contribute to an overly stimulating atmosphere. Soft, muted colours enhance the Yin quality of the space, fostering a serene and rejuvenating environment.

Plants and Natural Elements:

Introduce elements of nature in the bathroom to counterbalance the Water element. Plants, natural materials, and artwork depicting serene landscapes contribute to a harmonious and rejuvenating atmosphere. These elements connect the bathroom to the broader natural world, promoting a sense of balance and well-being.

Symbolic Imagery:

Incorporate symbols of purification and cleanliness in the bathroom. Artwork or decor featuring images of flowing water, clear skies, or cleansing elements evoke a sense of tranquility and purification. These symbols align with the intended purpose of the bathroom as a space for renewal and well-being.

Mindful Furniture and Decor Choices for Health and Wellness

Incorporating Feng Shui principles into the selection of furniture and decor further enhances the health-conscious atmosphere of your living spaces:

Furniture Choices:

opt for furniture with ergonomic designs that prioritize comfort and support. Choose pieces with natural materials and avoid those with sharp edges, which can create harsh energy. Consider the size and placement of furniture to maintain a balanced flow of Qi in each room.

Artwork and Decor:

Select artwork and decor that resonate with positive energy and contribute to a sense of well-being. Images of nature, serene landscapes, and symbols associated with health and vitality enhance the overall atmosphere. Be mindful of the symbolism and energy that each piece brings into your living spaces.

Textiles and Fabrics:

Soft, natural textiles contribute to a cosy and inviting atmosphere. Choose fabrics made from natural fibres, such as cotton or linen, for bedding, curtains, and upholstery. Introduce textures that feel nurturing and comforting, promoting a sense of well-being and relaxation.

Air-Purifying Plants:

Indoor plants not only contribute to better air quality but also bring the vibrant energy of nature indoors. Choose air-purifying plants such as snake plants, peace lilies, or spider plants to enhance the overall health-conscious environment. Be mindful of the specific needs of each plant and place them strategically in areas that could benefit from increased vitality.

Personalized Symbols for Health and Wellness:

Beyond the general Feng Shui principles, the integration of personalized symbols adds a layer of intention and meaning to your living spaces:

Symbols of Balance:

Incorporate symbols that represent balance and harmony. Yin-Yang symbols, mandalas, or representations of the Tai Chi symbol can serve as reminders to cultivate equilibrium in all aspects of life. Place these symbols in areas associated with health and well-being, reinforcing the intention for balance.

Personal Affirmations:

Infuse your living spaces with personal affirmations related to health and wellness. Create written affirmations that resonate with your goals and aspirations for well-being. Display them in areas where you can see and contemplate them regularly, fostering a positive mindset and promoting overall health.

Images of Inspirational Figures:

Display images or representations of figures who inspire you in the realm of health and wellness. This could include spiritual leaders, wellness practitioners, or individuals whose journeys resonate with your own health goals. Surrounding yourself with these images creates a supportive and motivating environment.

Vision Boards:

Craft a vision board that visually represents your health and wellness goals. Include images, words, and symbols that embody the vibrant and healthy life you aspire to lead. Place the vision board in a prominent location, such as the bedroom or a dedicated wellness space, to reinforce your intentions and attract positive energy.

Creating a Personalized Wellness Sanctuary: Case Studies

To illustrate the transformative power of Feng Shui in promoting health and wellness, let's explore two case studies where intentional adjustments were made to create personalized wellness sanctuaries:

Case Study 1: Restorative Bedroom Transformation

Challenge: A couple sought to transform their bedroom into a restful and rejuvenating sanctuary.

Solution: By adjusting the bed placement for optimal Qi flow, incorporating calming colours and textures, and introducing symbols of love and relaxation, the bedroom became a harmonious space that supported restful sleep and overall well-being.

Case Study 2: Energizing Kitchen Renovation

Challenge: A family aimed to revitalize their kitchen to promote healthier eating habits.

Solution: The kitchen layout was reorganized to enhance efficiency and flow. Vibrant colours and elements associated with nourishment were integrated, and symbols of abundance were strategically placed. These adjustments contributed to a revitalized kitchen that inspired healthier cooking and dining habits.

In the exploration of Feng Shui for health and wellness, we discover a profound synergy between our living spaces and the well-being of mind, body, and spirit. The intentional alignment of furniture, the mindful selection of colours, and the infusion of personalized symbols create an environment that supports balance, vitality, and harmony.

As we continue our journey into the realm of Feng Shui, let the principles discussed in this chapter serve as a guide to cultivate a living sanctuary that nurtures your health and wellness. From the restful embrace of your bedroom to the nourishing atmosphere of your kitchen, every corner of your home becomes an opportunity to enhance the quality of your life.

In the upcoming chapters, we will delve deeper into specific applications of Feng Shui, exploring advanced techniques, case studies, and real-life examples that highlight the profound impact of aligning our living spaces with the principles of harmony and well-being. So, with the wisdom of Feng Shui as our compass, let us continue this transformative journey toward a life of vibrant health and holistic wellness.

Chapter 6: Wealth and Prosperity in Feng Shui: Cultivating Abundance and Harmonizing Energy

In the intricate philosophy of Feng Shui, the pursuit of wealth and prosperity is seen as a harmonious dance between energy, intention, and the design of our living spaces. Chapter 6 embarks on a journey into the art of cultivating prosperity energy through the principles of Feng Shui. From the alignment of key areas to the careful selection of symbols and colours, every element within our environments plays a vital role in attracting wealth, opportunities, and a flow of abundance. In this chapter, we explore the profound ways in which Feng Shui can be harnessed to create an environment that resonates with prosperity.

The Essence of Prosperity in Feng Shui

At its core, Feng Shui views prosperity not only as material wealth but as the harmonious flow of energy that brings abundance in various aspects of life. Wealth, in the context of Feng Shui, encompasses financial stability, opportunities for growth, and the overall well-being of individuals and their families. The practice involves aligning the energy in our living spaces to create an environment that supports the manifestation of prosperity.

The Bagua Map: Mapping the Path to Prosperity

The Bagua Map, introduced earlier in Chapter 3, serves as a valuable guide in understanding the specific areas of our homes associated with prosperity. The Wealth gua, residing in the southeast quadrant of the Bagua, becomes the focal point for activating and enhancing prosperity energy.

Activating the Wealth Gua:

To activate the Wealth gua, direct your attention to the southeast area of your home or individual rooms. Introduce elements, colours, and symbols associated with prosperity to amplify the energy in this key zone. This may include the use of shades of purple or red, the incorporation of wealth symbols, and the strategic placement of items that represent abundance.

Water Element and Prosperity:

In Feng Shui, the Water element is closely tied to wealth and prosperity. Integrating water features, such as a fountain or aquarium, in the southeast area symbolizes the flow of abundance. It is crucial to keep these features clean and well-maintained, signifying the continuous influx of wealth.

Colour Choices for Prosperity:

Colours play a significant role in Feng Shui, each associated with specific elements and energies. For areas related to prosperity, incorporating auspicious colours is key. Hues of purple, red, and green are particularly favourable. These colours not only activate the Wealth gua but also resonate with the vibrant energy of abundance.

Enhancing Wealth with Symbols:

Introducing symbols of wealth and prosperity enhances the energy in designated areas. Consider incorporating objects like wealth vases, money plants, or wealth bowls adorned with symbols of abundance.

These items serve as powerful reminders of your financial goals and aspirations.

Maintaining Order and Clarity:

The Wealth gua thrives in an environment of order and clarity. Decluttering and organizing the southeast area contribute to the smooth flow of Qi, creating a space where prosperity energy can gather and circulate freely. A well-maintained and clutter-free environment aligns with the principles of Feng Shui, supporting the manifestation of wealth.

The Power of the Stove: Symbolism and Wealth in the Kitchen

In Feng Shui, the kitchen is regarded as the heart of the home, a space where the energies of nourishment and prosperity converge. Understanding the symbolic significance of the stove within the kitchen contributes to the cultivation of wealth energy.

Stove Placement and Wealth:

The stove holds a prominent place in Feng Shui, symbolizing both wealth and well-being. Placing the stove in a commanding position, allowing the cook to have a clear view of the kitchen entrance, is considered auspicious. This arrangement represents control and security, fostering a positive environment for the flow of abundance.

Well-Maintained Stove:

Keeping the stove in good working condition is symbolic of the continuous and steady flow of prosperity. A well-maintained stove aligns with the intention of creating a thriving and abundant atmosphere in the kitchen. Regular cleaning and repairs contribute to the overall harmony of the space.

Colours and Elements:

Infusing the kitchen with colours associated with prosperity enhances the wealth energy. Consider incorporating shades of green, yellow, or red in the kitchen decor. Elements of the Wood element, such as wooden utensils and cutting boards, contribute to the natural and vibrant energy associated with prosperity.

Abundance Symbols in the Kitchen:

Introducing symbols of abundance and prosperity in the kitchen reinforces the energy of wealth. Display items such as bowls of fresh fruit, symbols of good fortune, or images representing abundance. These symbols serve as daily reminders of the intention to attract prosperity through nourishment and sustenance.

Wealth Symbols and Their Significance

Feng Shui incorporates a variety of symbols believed to attract wealth and prosperity. Understanding the significance of these symbols allows for intentional placement within the home to amplify the energy of abundance.

The Money Tree:

The Money Tree, often associated with the Jade Plant or Pachira Aquatica, is a popular Feng Shui symbol of wealth and prosperity. Its rounded leaves are thought to resemble coins, making it a powerful symbol for inviting financial abundance. Placing a Money

Tree in the southeast corner of your living room or home office enhances the energy of prosperity.

The Wealth Vase:

The Wealth Vase is a traditional Feng Shui remedy believed to attract and accumulate wealth. It is a symbolic container filled with items that represent prosperity, such as precious stones, coins, and other auspicious objects. Placing a Wealth Vase in the southeast corner of your home or on your altar is believed to activate the flow of wealth energy.

The Laughing Buddha:

The Laughing Buddha, a well-known symbol in Chinese culture, is associated with happiness, wealth, and prosperity. Placing a Laughing Buddha statue in the southeast corner of your living room or workplace is believed to invite positive energy and financial success. The Buddha's joyful presence is thought to radiate good fortune and abundance.

The Wealth Bowl:

A Wealth Bowl is a symbolic container filled with precious stones, crystals, and other items associated with wealth. Creating a Wealth Bowl and placing it in the southeast corner of your home or on your work desk is believed to attract abundance and prosperity. The intentional selection of items in the bowl reinforces the energy of affluence.

The Three-Legged Toad (Chan Chu):

The Three-Legged Toad, also known as Chan Chu, is a popular Feng Shui symbol for wealth and prosperity. It is often depicted with a coin in its mouth, symbolizing the bringing of wealth into the home. Placing a Three-Legged Toad near the entrance of your home, facing inward, is believed to invite financial abundance and good fortune.

Water Features and the Flow of Prosperity Energy

In Feng Shui, water features are powerful symbols of abundance and prosperity. The sound and movement of water are associated with the flow of wealth energy, and incorporating water features strategically can enhance the prosperity in your living spaces.

Fountains and Aquariums:

Fountains and aquariums are popular water features used in Feng Shui to activate wealth energy. The continuous flow of water is symbolic of the steady influx of prosperity. Placing a fountain in the southeast corner of your garden or an aquarium in the southeast area of your living room invites the energy of abundance.

Mirrors and Water:

Mirrors strategically placed to reflect water features amplify the impact of water in Feng Shui. The combination of mirrors and water is believed to magnify the flow of prosperity energy. Consider placing a mirror behind a tabletop fountain or near an aquarium to enhance the visual presence of water in your space.

Caring for Water Features:

It is crucial to keep water features well-maintained to ensure the free flow of prosperity energy. Stagnant or dirty water can symbolize blocked or impeded wealth. Regular cleaning, proper filtration, and ensuring that water features are in good working condition contribute to the positive energy associated with prosperity.

Colours and Elements for Prosperity

Colours play a pivotal role in Feng Shui, with each colour corresponding to specific elements and energies. When cultivating wealth and prosperity, strategic use of colours associated with abundance enhances the overall energy flow.

Shades of Purple:

Purple is a colour often associated with wealth and abundance in Feng Shui. It is believed to activate the Wealth gua and stimulate the flow of prosperity energy. Incorporate shades of purple in your decor, such as throw pillows, artwork, or accents, to amplify the energy of abundance in designated areas.

Red and Gold Accents:

Red is considered an auspicious colour in Chinese culture and Feng Shui. It symbolizes good fortune, prosperity, and joy. Incorporate red accents in your decor, such as candles, artwork, or textiles, to invigorate the energy of wealth. Gold accents, associated with wealth and luxury, complement red and further enhance the auspicious energy.

Green for Growth:

Green, representing the Wood element, is associated with growth and vitality. Introducing shades of green in the southeast area of your home or in specific rooms amplifies the energy of prosperity. Consider using green plants, artwork, or decor to symbolize the flourishing of wealth and abundance.

Wooden Elements:

The Wood element is connected to prosperity and growth in Feng Shui. Incorporate wooden elements, such as furniture or decor made of wood, in the southeast area to enhance the energy of abundance. Wooden items symbolize the strength and resilience needed for financial success.

Earth Tones:

Earth tones, such as browns and yellows, are associated with stability and grounded energy. Introducing earthy colours in the southeast area creates a supportive environment for the manifestation of wealth. Use earth tones in furniture, textiles, or decor to anchor the energy of prosperity.

Personalized Affirmations for Wealth and Abundance:

In addition to external symbols and adjustments, incorporating personal affirmations aligned with wealth and abundance reinforces the intention to attract prosperity. Crafting and repeating positive statements related to financial well-being can have a powerful impact on the energy within your living spaces.

Creating Affirmation Statements:

Craft personalized affirmations that resonate with your financial goals and aspirations. Focus on statements that reflect abundance, prosperity, and financial success. For example, "I am open to receiving wealth and abundance in all areas of my life" or "Opportunities for prosperity flow to me effortlessly."

Displaying Affirmations:

Write or print your affirmation statements and display them in areas associated with prosperity. Place them on a vision board in the southeast corner of your living room or workspace. Creating a dedicated space for affirmations reinforces the positive energy of wealth and abundance.

Case Studies: Transformative Prosperity Alignments

To illustrate the transformative power of Feng Shui in cultivating wealth and prosperity, let's explore two case studies where intentional adjustments were made to create environments aligned with abundance:

Case Study 1: Activating Wealth in a Home Office

Challenge: A professional working from home sought to enhance financial opportunities and success in their career.

Solution: By activating the Wealth gua in the home office, incorporating symbols of abundance, and using colours associated with prosperity, the individual experienced a noticeable increase in financial opportunities, career growth, and overall abundance.

Case Study 2: Creating a Prosperity-Focused Living Room

Challenge: A family aimed to create a living room that supported financial prosperity and well-being.

Solution: Through strategic placement of symbols, such as a Wealth Vase and Money Tree, along with the use of auspicious colours, the family witnessed a positive shift in their financial situation. The living room became a space where the energy of wealth and abundance flourished.

As we conclude our exploration of Chapter 6, we've unveiled the intricacies of attracting wealth and abundance through the lens of Feng Shui. From activating the Wealth gua and incorporating symbols of prosperity to using specific colours and elements strategically, every adjustment contributes to the harmonization of energy that supports financial well-being.

Armed with the wisdom of Feng Shui, you now possess the knowledge to infuse your living spaces with prosperity energy. Whether it's the deliberate arrangement of symbols, the mindful use of colours, or the incorporation of personalized affirmations, each element plays a vital role in creating an environment that resonates with abundance.

In the forthcoming chapters, we will continue our exploration of Feng Shui, delving into advanced techniques, case studies, and practical applications that further illuminate the transformative power of this ancient practice. So, with the principles of prosperity in your toolkit, let the journey toward a life of abundance and financial well-being continue, guided by the timeless wisdom of Feng Shui.

Chapter 7: Love and Relationships in Feng Shui: Nurturing Harmonious Connections

In the intricate tapestry of Feng Shui, the energy that flows through our living spaces profoundly influences not only our individual well-being but also the dynamics of our relationships. Chapter 7 embarks on a journey into the realm of love and relationships within the context of Feng Shui. By understanding the principles of energy flow, symbolism, and intentional design, we unravel the secrets to creating environments that nurture and enhance the connections we share with our loved ones. From the arrangement of furniture to the strategic use of colours and symbols, every element within our homes plays a pivotal role in fostering harmonious relationships.

The Foundations of Love and Relationships in Feng Shui

Feng Shui approaches relationships with a holistic perspective, recognizing that the energy within our living spaces directly impacts the quality of connections we share with others. Whether it's a romantic partnership, familial bonds, or friendships, the principles of Feng Shui offer guidance on creating an environment that supports love, communication, and understanding.

The Bagua Map: Mapping Love and Relationship Energy

As introduced in earlier chapters, the Bagua Map serves as a foundational tool in Feng Shui, guiding us to understand the specific areas of our homes associated with love and relationships. The Love and Marriage gua, typically located in the southwest quadrant of the Bagua, becomes the focal point for activating and enhancing the energy of love within our living spaces.

Activating the Love and Marriage Gua:

To activate the Love and Marriage gua, direct your attention to the southwest area of your home or individual rooms. Introduce elements, colours, and symbols associated with love and romance to amplify the energy in this key zone. This may involve using shades of pink or red, incorporating symbols of love, and placing items that evoke a sense of romance.

Symbolism of Love:

Symbols play a significant role in Feng Shui, and when it comes to love and relationships, intentional use of symbols can enhance the energy within a space. Items such as pairs of objects, artwork depicting loving scenes, or symbols of partnership contribute to the harmonious atmosphere in areas associated with love.

Enhancing Yin Energy:

The Love and Marriage gua is associated with Yin energy, which is receptive, nurturing, and represents the feminine aspect. Enhance Yin energy by incorporating soft textures, gentle lighting, and decor that exudes a sense of warmth and comfort. Creating a space that embraces Yin qualities contributes to the overall harmony of relationships.

Clutter Clearance:

As in other areas of Feng Shui, clutter is considered an obstacle to the free flow of energy. Decluttering and organizing the southwest area of your home create a space where love energy can circulate freely. Remove any items that evoke negative emotions or memories, allowing the energy of love to thrive.

The Bedroom: A Sanctuary for Love and Intimacy

In Feng Shui, the bedroom holds special significance as a sanctuary for love, intimacy, and connection. Creating an environment that supports the romantic aspect of relationships involves intentional adjustments and thoughtful design choices.

Bed Placement:

The placement of the bed is a crucial consideration in Feng Shui for the bedroom. Position the bed in a commanding position, allowing a clear view of the bedroom entrance while avoiding direct alignment with it. This arrangement enhances a sense of security and openness, fostering a positive atmosphere for love and intimacy.

Colours of Romance:

The choice of colours in the bedroom sets the tone for the romantic energy. Soft and muted tones, such as shades of pink, red, and warm neutrals, create a romantic and inviting ambiance. These colours resonate with the energy of love and passion, contributing to a harmonious atmosphere.

Balancing Yin and Yang:

Striking a balance between Yin and Yang energies is crucial in the bedroom. Soft textures, gentle lighting, and romantic decor contribute to Yin qualities, creating a nurturing and intimate space. Maintain a sense of order and cleanliness to infuse Yang qualities, promoting a harmonious balance between restful sleep and romantic connection.

Personalized Symbols of Love:

Infusing the bedroom with symbols of love enhances the romantic energy. Consider incorporating items such as artwork depicting romantic scenes, pairs of objects symbolizing partnership, or meaningful mementos that evoke positive emotions. These symbols serve as visual reminders of the love shared within the space.

The Living Room: Fostering Harmonious Connections

The living room, being a central gathering space for family and friends, plays a significant role in nurturing harmonious relationships. Applying Feng Shui principles to this shared area involves intentional design choices that promote communication, connection, and a sense of unity.

Seating Arrangement:

The arrangement of furniture in the living room affects the dynamics of communication and connection. Position sofas and chairs in a way that encourages face-to-face interaction, creating a conducive environment for conversations and shared experiences. Avoid placing furniture in a way that creates barriers or obstacles to communication.

Harmonious Colours:

Colours in the living room influence the overall energy of the space. Choose colours that promote harmony and connection, such as warm neutrals, soft blues, or earthy tones. Avoid overly vibrant or conflicting colours that may create tension. The goal is to create a welcoming and inviting atmosphere that supports positive interactions.

Personalized Symbols:

Personalize the living room with symbols that represent family unity and connection. Display family photographs, artwork created by family members, or items that hold sentimental value. These personalized symbols contribute to a sense of belonging and strengthen the bonds between family members.

Artwork and Decor:

Select artwork and decor that resonates with positive emotions and shared interests. Images of nature, scenes depicting joy and togetherness, or symbols of unity create an uplifting atmosphere. Be mindful of the symbolism and energy that each piece brings into the living room, ensuring that it aligns with the intention of fostering harmonious connections.

The Dining Area: Nourishing Relationships

The dining area serves as a space where families and friends come together to share meals and connect. Feng Shui principles applied to the dining area focus on creating an environment that fosters nourishment, communication, and a sense of unity.

Table Placement:

The placement of the dining table is significant in Feng Shui. Position the table in a way that allows everyone to have a clear view of the room's entrance. This arrangement promotes a sense of inclusivity and unity during meals. Avoid placing the dining table directly in line with the door, as it may create a disruptive energy flow.

Balancing Yin and Yang:

Balance the energy in the dining area by incorporating both Yin and Yang qualities. Soft lighting, comfortable seating, and elements of warmth contribute to Yin energy, creating a nurturing and inviting space. Maintain order and cleanliness to infuse Yang qualities, promoting a harmonious atmosphere for shared meals.

Colours for Connection:

Choose colours for the dining area that evoke a sense of connection and togetherness. Warm tones, such as earthy browns and soft yellows, create a welcoming ambiance. Consider using table linens, placemats, or decor in colours that align with the intention of fostering positive connections during meals.

Symbolic Centrepiece:

The centrepiece on the dining table can serve as a symbolic focal point. Choose items that symbolize unity, abundance, and nourishment. A bowl of fresh fruit, a vase of flowers, or a meaningful centrepiece can enhance the energy of the dining area, creating an atmosphere conducive to positive interactions.

Personalized Symbols for Love and Relationships:

Beyond the general Feng Shui principles, the integration of personalized symbols adds a layer of intention and meaning to your living spaces.

Couples' Symbols:

Infuse your home with symbols that represent the partnership and connection between couples. This could include artwork or decor featuring pairs of objects, symbols of love and unity, or items that hold sentimental value to both partners. These symbols strengthen the bond between couples and contribute to a harmonious living environment.

Family Crests or Emblems:

Consider creating a family crest or emblem that represents the values and unity of your family. Display this emblem in a prominent location, such as the entrance or a shared living space. The family crest becomes a symbol of identity and fosters a sense of belonging and togetherness.

Intentional Artwork:

Choose artwork that reflects the energy you want to cultivate in your relationships. Images of happy families, scenes of togetherness, or symbols of love can be strategically placed in areas associated with relationships. The intentional selection of artwork reinforces the positive energy of love and connection.

Personalized Altar or Shrine:

Create a personalized altar or shrine dedicated to the energy of love and relationships. Include items that hold sentimental value, such as photos, mementos, or symbolic objects representing love. This sacred space becomes a focal point for intentional connection and serves as a reminder of the love shared within the home.

Case Studies: Transformative Relationship Alignments

To illustrate the transformative power of Feng Shui in enhancing love and relationships, let's explore two case studies where intentional adjustments were made to create environments aligned with harmonious connections:

Case Study 1: Revitalizing a Romantic Bedroom

Challenge: A couple sought to rekindle the romance and intimacy in their relationship.

Solution: By applying Feng Shui principles to the bedroom, including strategic bed placement, romantic colours, and personalized symbols of love, the couple experienced a noticeable improvement in their connection. The bedroom became a sanctuary that supported both restful sleep and romantic intimacy.

Case Study 2: Fostering Family Unity in the Living Room

Challenge: A family aimed to create a living room that promoted positive interactions and unity.

Solution: Through intentional furniture arrangement, harmonious colours, and personalized symbols of family connection, the living room became a space where family members felt a stronger sense of togetherness. Positive interactions increased, fostering a more cohesive and supportive family environment.

As we conclude our exploration of Chapter 7, the principles of Feng Shui reveal the profound impact of intentional design on the dynamics of love and relationships within our homes. From activating the Love and Marriage gua to creating harmonious spaces in the bedroom, living room, and dining area, every adjustment contributes to the cultivation of positive energy.

Armed with the wisdom of Feng Shui, you now possess the tools to infuse your living spaces with love and harmony. Whether it's the deliberate arrangement of furniture, the mindful selection of colours, or the incorporation of personalized symbols, each element plays a crucial role in creating an environment that nurtures and enhances the connections you share with your loved ones.

In the upcoming chapters, we will continue our exploration of Feng Shui, delving into advanced techniques, case studies, and practical applications that further illuminate the transformative power of this ancient practice. So, with the principles of love and relationships as your guide, let the journey toward harmonious connections within your home and heart continue, guided by the timeless wisdom of Feng Shui.

Chapter 8: Career and Success in Feng Shui: Cultivating Professional Prosperity

In the intricate landscape of Feng Shui, the energy that permeates our living and working spaces significantly influences our career trajectory and overall success. Chapter 8 embarks on an exploration of the principles and practices within Feng Shui that guide us in cultivating professional prosperity. From the strategic arrangement of workspaces to the intentional use of symbols and colours, every element within our environments plays a crucial role in aligning our careers with the principles of harmony and success.

Foundations of Career and Success in Feng Shui

Feng Shui approaches the concept of career and success with a holistic perspective, acknowledging the interconnectedness between our professional lives and the energy within our surroundings. By understanding the flow of energy, harnessing auspicious symbols, and making intentional design choices, individuals can create environments that support career growth, opportunities, and overall success.

The Bagua Map: Mapping the Path to Professional Prosperity

As introduced in previous chapters, the Bagua Map serves as a fundamental guide in Feng Shui, helping us identify specific areas of our homes and offices associated with career and success. The Career gua, located in the north sector of the Bagua, becomes the focal point for activating and enhancing the energy of career and professional advancement.

Activating the Career Gua:

To activate the Career gua, focus on the north sector of your home or individual rooms. Introduce elements, colours, and symbols associated with career success to amplify the energy in this key zone. This may involve using shades of black or deep blue, incorporating symbols of career growth, and placing items that evoke a sense of professionalism and accomplishment.

Water Element and Career Success:

In Feng Shui, the Water element is closely tied to career success and the flow of opportunities. Integrating water features, such as a tabletop fountain or an aquarium, in the north area symbolizes the steady influx of opportunities and the smooth progression of one's career. It is essential to keep these features clean and well-maintained to signify continuous growth.

Colour Choices for Career Prosperity:

Colours play a pivotal role in Feng Shui, each associated with specific elements and energies. For areas related to career and success, incorporating auspicious colours is key. Hues of black, deep blue, and white are particularly favourable. These colours not only activate the Career gua but also resonate with the energy of professionalism and achievement.

Enhancing Career with Symbols:

Introducing symbols of career success enhances the energy in designated areas. Consider incorporating objects like a career vision board, a desk ornament representing your profession, or symbols associated with advancement and recognition. These items serve as powerful reminders of your professional goals and aspirations.

The Office: Designing a Workspace for Success

The design and arrangement of the office play a crucial role in fostering a productive and successful work environment. Applying Feng Shui principles to the office involves intentional adjustments and thoughtful design choices that promote career growth and overall success.

Desk Placement:

The placement of the desk is a critical consideration in Feng Shui for the office. Position the desk in a commanding position, allowing a clear view of the office entrance while avoiding direct alignment with it. This arrangement enhances a sense of control, authority, and openness, fostering a positive atmosphere for career success.

Colours for Professionalism:

The choice of colours in the office sets the tone for a professional and success-oriented environment. Neutral tones, such as shades of white, beige, or light Gray, create a clean and organized atmosphere. Incorporate accents of black or deep blue to activate the energy of the Career gua and stimulate professional achievement.

Organizational Strategies:

Organization is paramount in the office environment. Declutter the workspace regularly and maintain a sense of order to allow the free flow of energy. A clutter-free environment not only enhances productivity but also aligns with Feng Shui principles, promoting success and career advancement.

Personalized Success Symbols:

Personalize the office with symbols that represent your professional aspirations and achievements. Display awards, certificates, or items that signify recognition for your work. These personalized symbols contribute to a motivational and success-driven atmosphere within the office.

The Entrance: Welcoming Opportunities

The entrance of the office serves as the first point of contact with the energy entering the space. Applying Feng Shui principles to the entrance involves creating a welcoming and inviting atmosphere that attracts opportunities and success.

Clear Pathways:

Ensure that pathways leading to the office entrance are clear and unobstructed. This allows the energy, or Qi, to flow smoothly into the space, bringing with it opportunities and positive vibrations. Remove any obstacles or clutter that may hinder the free flow of energy.

Welcoming Colours:

Choose welcoming colours for the entrance that align with the energy of success. Warm and inviting tones, such as shades of gold, red, or green, create a positive first impression. Consider incorporating these colours in the entrance decor or signage to evoke a sense of professionalism and success.

Symbolic Signage:

Utilize symbolic signage or decor at the entrance that represents success and prosperity. Incorporate symbols associated with achievements, such as a depiction of a mountain (symbolizing stability and career advancement) or the image of a key (symbolizing unlocking opportunities). These symbols set the tone for success from the moment individuals enter the office.

Water Features and Career Advancement

Water features hold special significance in Feng Shui for career success. The inclusion of water elements, such as fountains or aquariums, strategically enhances the energy of career advancement and opportunity.

Fountains for Prosperity:

Indoor fountains, placed in the north area of the office, symbolize the flow of opportunities and career advancement. The sound and movement of water are associated with prosperity, and a well-maintained fountain serves as a powerful symbol of success. Choose a fountain with a design that complements the overall decor of the office.

Aquariums for Flowing Energy:

Aquariums, with their flowing water and vibrant aquatic life, are considered auspicious for career success. Place an aquarium in the north sector of the office to symbolize the continuous flow of opportunities. Ensure that the aquarium is clean, well-maintained, and positioned in a way that aligns with Feng Shui principles.

Mirrors and Water:

Mirrors strategically placed to reflect water features amplify the impact of water in Feng Shui. The combination of mirrors and water is believed to magnify the flow of career energy. Consider placing a mirror near a tabletop fountain or an aquarium to enhance the visual presence of water in your workspace.

Colours and Elements for Professional Success

Colours and elements play a pivotal role in Feng Shui, and their strategic use in the office environment can enhance the energy of professional success.

Black and Deep Blue:

Black and deep blue are colours associated with the Water element and are considered auspicious for career success. Incorporate these colours in the office decor, such as in furniture, accents, or artwork, to activate the energy of the Career gua. These colours convey a sense of professionalism, authority, and accomplishment.

Metal Element:

The Metal element is associated with precision, focus, and success in Feng Shui. Introduce metal elements in the office through decor, such as metallic accents, office supplies made of metal, or artwork featuring metal structures. The Metal element enhances the energy of clarity and precision, contributing to career advancement.

Crystal and Glass Decor:

Crystal and glass elements represent the Water element in Feng Shui and are believed to enhance career success. Incorporate crystal or glass decor in the office, such as paperweights, desk accessories, or artwork. The transparent and reflective nature of these materials aligns with the energy of clarity and focus on professional endeavours.

Wood Element for Growth:

The Wood element symbolizes growth and upward movement, making it conducive to career advancement. Introduce wooden elements in the office through furniture, decor, or plants. Wooden items represent the energy of resilience and growth, fostering an environment that supports professional development.

Personalized Success Affirmations:

In addition to external adjustments, incorporating personalized affirmations aligned with career success reinforces the intention to attract professional opportunities. Crafting and repeating positive statements related to career advancement can have a powerful impact on the energy within your workspace.

Crafting Affirmation Statements:

Create personalized affirmations that resonate with your career goals and aspirations. Focus on statements that reflect success, achievement, and continuous growth. For example, "I am open to receiving new opportunities and advancements in my career" or "I attract success and prosperity in all my professional endeavours."

Displaying Affirmations:

Write or print your affirmation statements and display them in the office. Place them on your desk, vision board, or in areas associated with the Career gua. Creating a dedicated space for affirmations reinforces the positive energy of professional success and serves as a daily reminder of your career goals.

Case Studies: Transformative Career Alignments

To illustrate the transformative power of Feng Shui in cultivating career success, let's explore two case studies where intentional adjustments were made to create environments aligned with professional prosperity:

Case Study 1: Elevating an Executive Office

Challenge: An executive seeking career advancement and increased opportunities wanted to enhance the energy in their office.

Solution: By applying Feng Shui principles, including strategic desk placement, incorporation of water elements, and use of colours associated with career success, the executive experienced a noticeable improvement in their career trajectory. Opportunities for advancement and recognition increased, aligning with the positive energy cultivated in the office.

Case Study 2: Transforming a Creative Workspace

Challenge: A creative professional wanted to infuse their workspace with energy that would support both creativity and career success.

Solution: By incorporating elements such as a tabletop fountain, personalized success symbols, and a balanced use of colours and elements, the creative professional witnessed a positive shift in their career. The workspace became a source of inspiration, fostering not only creative endeavours but also attracting opportunities for professional growth.

As we conclude our exploration of Chapter 8, the principles of Feng Shui unveil the profound impact of intentional design on the dynamics of career and success within our professional spaces. From activating the Career gua to creating a conducive office environment, every adjustment contributes to the cultivation of positive energy that supports professional growth.

Armed with the wisdom of Feng Shui, you now possess the tools to infuse your workspace with the energy of career success. Whether it's the deliberate arrangement of the office layout, the mindful selection of colours, or the incorporation of personalized symbols, each element plays a crucial role in creating an environment that propels your career forward.

In the forthcoming chapters, we will continue our exploration of Feng Shui, delving into advanced techniques, case studies, and practical applications that further illuminate the transformative power of this ancient practice. So, with the principles of career and success as your guide, let the journey toward professional prosperity continue, guided by the timeless wisdom of Feng Shui.

Chapter 9: Feng Shui for Family Harmony: Creating a Haven of Unity

In the intricate tapestry of Feng Shui, the energy that circulates within our homes profoundly influences the dynamics of family life. Chapter 9 embarks on an exploration of the principles and practices within Feng Shui that guide us in fostering family harmony. By understanding the flow of energy, harnessing auspicious symbols, and making intentional design choices, individuals can create environments that support unity, communication, and overall well-being within the family unit.

Foundations of Family Harmony in Feng Shui

Feng Shui views the family as a vital unit within the home, recognizing the interconnectedness between individuals and the energy circulating within shared spaces. The principles of family harmony in Feng Shui aim to create an environment that nurtures positive relationships, open communication, and a sense of togetherness.

The Bagua Map: Navigating Family Connections

As established in earlier chapters, the Bagua Map is a foundational tool in Feng Shui, guiding us to understand the specific areas of our homes associated with family harmony. The Family gua, typically located in the east sector of the Bagua, becomes the focal point for activating and enhancing the energy of familial connections.

Activating the Family Gua:

To activate the Family gua, focus on the east sector of your home or individual rooms. Introduce elements, colours, and symbols associated with family unity to amplify the energy in this key zone. This may involve using shades of green or brown, incorporating symbols of family love, and placing items that evoke a sense of togetherness.

Wood Element for Growth:

In Feng Shui, the Wood element is associated with family growth and vitality. Introduce wooden elements in the east area through furniture, decor, or plants. Wooden items symbolize the strength and resilience needed for family well-being, fostering an environment that supports growth and positive connections.

Colour Choices for Family Unity:

Colours play a crucial role in Feng Shui, each associated with specific elements and energies. For areas related to family harmony, incorporating auspicious colours is key. Hues of green and brown are particularly favourable. These colours not only activate the Family gua but also resonate with the energy of growth, balance, and unity.

Symbolism of Family Love:

Introducing symbols of family love enhances the energy in designated areas. Consider incorporating items such as family portraits, artwork depicting harmonious scenes, or symbols representing unity. These symbols serve as powerful reminders of the love and connection shared within the family.

The Living Room: Fostering Togetherness

The living room, being a central gathering space for family members, plays a significant role in nurturing family harmony. Applying Feng Shui principles to this shared area involves intentional design choices that promote communication, connection, and a sense of unity.

Seating Arrangement:

The arrangement of furniture in the living room affects the dynamics of family interactions. Position sofas and chairs in a way that encourages face-to-face interaction, creating a conducive environment for conversations and shared experiences. Avoid placing furniture in a way that creates barriers or obstacles to communication.

Harmonious Colours:

Colours in the living room influence the overall energy of the space. Choose colours that promote harmony and connection, such as warm neutrals, soft blues, or earthy tones. Avoid overly vibrant or conflicting colours that may create tension. The goal is to create a welcoming and inviting atmosphere that supports positive interactions.

Personalized Symbols:

Personalize the living room with symbols that represent family unity. Display family photographs, artwork created by family members, or items that hold sentimental value. These personalized symbols contribute to a sense of belonging and strengthen the bonds between family members.

Family Altar or Shrine:

Create a family altar or shrine in the living room dedicated to the energy of family harmony. Include items that symbolize love, unity, and positive connections. This sacred space becomes a focal point for intentional family gatherings and serves as a reminder of the love and support shared within the home.

The Dining Area: Nurturing Family Connections

The dining area serves as a space where families come together to share meals and connect. Feng Shui principles applied to the dining area focus on creating an environment that fosters nourishment, communication, and a sense of unity.

Table Placement:

The placement of the dining table is significant in Feng Shui. Position the table in a way that allows everyone to have a clear view of the room's entrance. This arrangement promotes a sense of inclusivity and unity during meals. Avoid placing the dining table directly in line with the door, as it may create a disruptive energy flow.

Balancing Yin and Yang:

Balance the energy in the dining area by incorporating both Yin and Yang qualities. Soft lighting, comfortable seating, and elements of warmth contribute to Yin energy, creating a nurturing and inviting space. Maintain order and cleanliness to infuse Yang qualities, promoting a harmonious atmosphere for shared meals.

Colours for Connection:

Choose colours for the dining area that evoke a sense of connection and togetherness. Warm tones, such as earthy browns and soft yellows, create a welcoming ambiance. Consider using table linens, placemats, or decor in colours that align with the intention of fostering positive connections during meals.

Symbolic Centrepiece:

The centrepiece on the dining table can serve as a symbolic focal point. Choose items that symbolize unity, abundance, and nourishment. A bowl of fresh fruit, a vase of flowers, or a meaningful centrepiece can enhance the energy of the dining area, creating an atmosphere conducive to positive interactions.

The Bedroom: Fostering Intimacy and Understanding

While the bedroom is often considered a private space, applying Feng Shui principles to this area contributes to the overall harmony of family relationships. The bedroom is where couples share their most intimate moments and where parents find solace. Creating an environment that fosters intimacy and understanding enhances the overall well-being of the family.

Bed Placement:

The placement of the bed is a crucial consideration in Feng Shui for the bedroom. Position the bed in a commanding position, allowing a clear view of the bedroom entrance while avoiding direct alignment with it. This arrangement enhances a sense of security and openness, fostering a positive atmosphere for family unity.

Colours for Serenity:

The choice of colours in the bedroom sets the tone for a serene and harmonious atmosphere. Soft and muted tones, such as shades of blue, green, or warm neutrals, create a tranquil ambiance. These colours resonate with the energy of relaxation and understanding, contributing to a harmonious family environment.

Balancing Yin and Yang:

Striking a balance between Yin and Yang energies is crucial in the bedroom. Soft textures, gentle lighting, and romantic decor contribute to Yin qualities, creating a nurturing and intimate space. Maintain a sense of order and cleanliness to infuse Yang qualities, promoting a harmonious balance between restful sleep and family connection.

Family Symbols in the Bedroom:

Infuse the bedroom with symbols that represent family unity and love. Display artwork or decor featuring images of family members, symbols of togetherness, or items that hold sentimental value. These symbols serve as visual reminders of the strong bonds shared within the family, creating a sense of security and connection.

Children's Rooms: Nurturing Growth and Harmony

Feng Shui principles can be applied to children's rooms to create environments that support their well-being, growth, and harmony within the family. From the layout of furniture to the choice of colours and decor, intentional design choices contribute to a positive and nurturing atmosphere.

Bed Placement and Study Areas:

Arrange the bed and study areas in a way that fosters a sense of security and concentration. Avoid placing the bed directly in line with the door and ensure that the study desk is positioned to minimize distractions. This arrangement contributes to a harmonious environment that supports both rest and focused learning.

Colours for Positive Energy:

Choose colours for children's rooms that evoke positive energy and creativity. Soft pastels, shades of green, or light blues create a soothing and uplifting atmosphere. Incorporate colours that align with the child's preferences and interests, allowing them to express their individuality within the space.

Personalized Symbols:

Personalize children's rooms with symbols that represent their interests and aspirations. Display artwork, decor, or items related to their hobbies, dreams, or favourite activities. Creating a space that reflects their personality fosters a sense of belonging and connection within the family.

Organization and Clutter Control:

Maintain an organized and clutter-free environment in children's rooms. Encourage the practice of tidying up and organizing belongings regularly. A well-organized space not only contributes to a harmonious atmosphere but also instils positive habits in children, promoting a sense of responsibility within the family.

Outdoor Spaces: Extending Harmony to Nature

Feng Shui principles can be extended to outdoor spaces, creating a harmonious connection between the family and nature. Whether it's a backyard, garden, or balcony, intentional design choices contribute to an environment that promotes relaxation, unity, and overall well-being.

Outdoor Seating Arrangements:

Arrange outdoor seating in a way that encourages family gatherings and conversations. Create a comfortable and inviting space with well-placed seating, cushions, and decor. Designate areas for relaxation and recreation, fostering a sense of togetherness in the outdoor environment.

Natural Elements and Plants:

Incorporate natural elements and plants in outdoor spaces to enhance the connection with nature. Choose plants with vibrant and positive energy, and strategically place them to create a harmonious flow. The presence of greenery contributes to a serene and refreshing atmosphere, promoting family well-being.

Symbolic Outdoor Decor:

Use symbolic outdoor decor to reinforce the energy of family harmony. Consider placing items such as statues or ornaments that represent unity, love, and growth. These symbolic elements contribute to a positive and uplifting outdoor environment, aligning with the principles of Feng Shui.

Case Studies: Transformative Family Alignments

To illustrate the transformative power of Feng Shui in fostering family harmony, let's explore two case studies where intentional adjustments were made to create environments aligned with positive connections:

Case Study 1: Cultivating Family Unity in the Living Room

Challenge: A family sought to enhance the sense of togetherness in their living room, fostering positive interactions and communication.

Solution: By applying Feng Shui principles, including strategic furniture arrangement, harmonious colours, and personalized symbols of family love, the living room became a space where family members felt a stronger sense of connection. Positive interactions increased, creating a harmonious and supportive family environment.

Case Study 2: Transforming Children's Rooms for Harmony

Challenge: Parents wanted to create bedrooms for their children that not only reflected their individuality but also contributed to overall family harmony.

Solution: Through intentional bed placement, the use of soothing colours, personalized symbols, and an organized environment, the children's rooms became spaces that nurtured both individual growth and family connections. The children felt a sense of ownership and belonging within the family unit.

As we conclude our exploration of Chapter 9, the principles of Feng Shui reveal the profound impact of intentional design on the dynamics of family harmony within our homes. From activating the

Family gua to creating harmonious spaces in shared areas, bedrooms, and outdoor environments, every adjustment contributes to the cultivation of positive energy that supports unity and well-being.

Armed with the wisdom of Feng Shui, you now possess the tools to infuse your living spaces with the energy of family harmony. Whether it's the deliberate arrangement of furniture, the mindful selection of colours, or the incorporation of personalized symbols, each element plays a crucial role in creating an environment that nurtures and enhances the connections within your family.

In the forthcoming chapters, we will continue our exploration of Feng Shui, delving into advanced techniques, case studies, and practical applications that further illuminate the transformative power of this ancient practice. So, with the principles of family harmony as your guide, let the journey toward creating a haven of unity within your home continue, guided by the timeless wisdom of Feng Shui.

Chapter 10: Enhancing Creativity and Knowledge in Feng Shui: Unleashing the Power of Mindful Spaces

In the rich tapestry of Feng Shui, the arrangement of our surroundings extends beyond the physical realm, influencing our mental clarity, creativity, and thirst for knowledge. Chapter 10 embarks on an exploration of the principles and practices within Feng Shui that guide us in enhancing creativity and knowledge. By understanding the flow of energy, incorporating auspicious symbols, and making intentional design choices, individuals can create environments that inspire innovative thinking, foster learning, and amplify the power of the mind.

Foundations of Creativity and Knowledge in Feng Shui

Feng Shui recognizes the interconnectedness between our physical spaces and the mental realms of creativity and knowledge. The principles guiding creativity and knowledge in Feng Shui are rooted in creating environments that stimulate mental agility, support focused learning, and cultivate a mindset of continuous curiosity.

The Bagua Map: Mapping the Path to Mental Prowess

As introduced in previous chapters, the Bagua Map serves as a guiding tool in Feng Shui, helping us identify specific areas of our homes associated with creativity and knowledge. The Knowledge and Wisdom gua, typically located in the northeast sector of the Bagua, becomes the focal point for activating and enhancing the energy of intellectual pursuits.

Activating the Knowledge Gua:

To activate the Knowledge gua, focus on the northeast sector of your home or individual rooms. Introduce elements, colours, and symbols associated with knowledge and wisdom to amplify the energy in this key zone. This may involve using shades of blue or black, incorporating symbols of scholarly pursuits, and placing items that evoke a sense of mental clarity.

Earth Element for Stability:

In Feng Shui, the Earth element is associated with stability and grounding, crucial for supporting intellectual endeavours. Introduce Earth elements in the northeast area through decor, such as clay pottery, stones, or earthy colours. These elements contribute to a stable and focused energy conducive to learning and creativity.

Colours for Intellectual Stimulation:

Colours play a pivotal role in Feng Shui, each associated with specific elements and energies. For areas related to creativity and knowledge, incorporating auspicious colours is key. Hues of blue and black are particularly favourable. These colours not only activate the Knowledge gua but also resonate with the energy of focus, concentration, and intellectual stimulation.

Symbolic Representation of Knowledge:

Introducing symbols associated with knowledge and learning enhances the energy in designated areas. Consider incorporating items such as books, educational tools, or symbols representing wisdom. These symbolic elements serve as visual cues that inspire a mindset of continuous learning and intellectual growth.

The Study or Home Office: Crafting a Haven for Creativity

The study or home office is a sanctuary where creativity and knowledge flourish. Applying Feng Shui principles to this space involves intentional design choices that promote concentration, innovative thinking, and a thirst for knowledge.

Desk Placement for Focus:

The placement of the desk is a critical consideration in Feng Shui for the study or home office. Position the desk in a way that allows a clear view of the room and entrance. This arrangement enhances a sense of control and openness, fostering a positive atmosphere for focused work, creativity, and learning.

Colours for Concentration:

Choose colours for the study or home office that promote concentration and mental clarity. Shades of blue, black, or deep Gray create a serene and focused ambiance. Avoid overly vibrant or distracting colours that may hinder concentration. The goal is to create a space that supports deep thought and innovative ideas.

Organizational Strategies:

Organization is paramount in the study or home office environment. Declutter the workspace regularly and maintain a sense of order to allow the free flow of energy. A well-organized space not only enhances productivity but also aligns with Feng Shui principles, promoting mental clarity and creativity.

Inspirational Symbols:

Infuse the study or home office with symbols that inspire creativity and knowledge. Display artwork, quotes, or items related to your field of interest or study. Personalizing the space with items that resonate with your passions and aspirations contributes to a motivational and inspiring atmosphere.

Creativity and Knowledge Corners: Designated Spaces for Inspiration

Designating specific corners or areas within your home to creativity and knowledge further enhances the energy conducive to innovative thinking and intellectual pursuits.

Creativity Corner:

Designate a corner in a common area or your personal space as a creativity corner. Introduce elements that stimulate creative thinking, such as artistic decor, inspirational quotes, or a vision board. This corner becomes a sacred space for brainstorming, ideation, and the cultivation of innovative ideas.

Knowledge Nook:

Create a knowledge nook in an area associated with the Knowledge gua. Place a bookshelf, desk, or comfortable reading chair along with items that symbolize learning and wisdom. This designated space becomes a haven for focused study, reading, and intellectual exploration.

Flexible Arrangements:

Keep in mind that Feng Shui is adaptable to individual preferences and needs. Whether it's a creativity corner in the living room or a knowledge nook in the bedroom, flexible arrangements allow you to tailor designated spaces to your unique requirements, fostering a harmonious blend of creativity and knowledge within your home.

Inspiration from Nature: Outdoor Spaces for Intellectual Reflection

Outdoor spaces can also serve as inspirational settings for intellectual reflection and creativity. Utilizing Feng Shui principles in outdoor environments contributes to a harmonious connection between nature and the mind.

Outdoor Reading Areas:

Create outdoor reading areas with comfortable seating, surrounded by nature. Position chairs or benches in a way that allows for unobstructed views, promoting a sense of openness and mental clarity. Incorporate elements such as potted plants, wind chimes, or symbolic decor to enhance the energy of intellectual pursuits.

Garden of Ideas:

Designate a portion of your garden or outdoor space as a "Garden of Ideas." Plant flowers, herbs, or trees that are associated with mental clarity and inspiration. Consider creating a labyrinth or meandering path for contemplative walks, allowing the mind to wander and generate creative thoughts.

Symbolic Outdoor Decor:

Use symbolic outdoor decor, such as sculptures or ornaments representing knowledge and creativity. Place these items strategically in outdoor spaces to serve as visual reminders of the intellectual pursuits that bring joy and fulfilment. The outdoor environment becomes an extension of your mindful spaces, supporting mental well-being.

Colours and Elements for Creative Energy

Colours and elements play a significant role in Feng Shui, and their strategic use in your environment can enhance the energy of creativity and knowledge.

Blue for Communication and Creativity:

Blue is a colour associated with the Water element, symbolizing communication, and creative expression. Incorporate shades of blue in areas where you engage in creative activities, such as writing, brainstorming, or artistic pursuits. Blue promotes a calming yet stimulating atmosphere conducive to innovative thinking.

Black for Wisdom and Depth:

Black is a colour associated with the Water element and represents wisdom and depth. Introduce black accents, such as decor or furniture, in spaces dedicated to knowledge and intellectual pursuits. Black adds a sense of sophistication and encourages introspection, creating an environment that supports deep thinking.

Metal Element for Clarity:

The Metal element is associated with clarity and precision in Feng Shui. Introduce metal elements in creative and study spaces through decor, such as metallic accents, frames, or sculptures. The presence of metal enhances mental clarity and sharpens focus, contributing to effective creative and learning environments.

Earth Element for Stability:

The Earth element provides stability and grounding, essential for fostering creativity and knowledge. Incorporate earthy colours, such as browns and yellows, in areas where you engage in intellectual pursuits. Earthy tones create a stable and nurturing atmosphere, supporting a grounded mindset for learning and creative exploration.

Personalized Affirmations for Creativity and Knowledge:

In addition to external adjustments, incorporating personalized affirmations aligned with creativity and knowledge reinforces the intention to expand your intellectual horizons.

Crafting Affirmation Statements:

Create personalized affirmations that resonate with your aspirations for creativity and knowledge. Focus on statements that reflect a mindset of continuous learning, inspiration, and innovative thinking. For example, "I am open to creative ideas that flow effortlessly" or "I am a lifelong learner, constantly expanding my knowledge."

Displaying Affirmations:

Write or print your affirmation statements and display them in areas associated with creativity and knowledge. Place them on your desk, in your creativity corner, or near your knowledge nook. Creating a dedicated space for affirmations reinforces the positive energy of intellectual pursuits and serves as a daily reminder of your commitment to creativity and learning.

Case Studies: Transformative Mindful Spaces

To illustrate the transformative power of Feng Shui in enhancing creativity and knowledge, let's explore two case studies where intentional adjustments were made to create environments aligned with intellectual pursuits:

Case Study 1: Transforming a Home Office for Creativity

Challenge: A professional working from home sought to infuse their home office with creativity and innovative thinking.

Solution: By applying Feng Shui principles, including strategic desk placement, incorporation of blue and black accents, and personalized symbols of inspiration, the home office became a dynamic space for creative work. The individual reported an increase in innovative ideas and a heightened sense of focus and clarity.

Case Study 2: Creating a Knowledge Nook for Lifelong Learning

Challenge: An avid reader and learner desired a dedicated space for focused study and intellectual exploration.

Solution: By designating a knowledge nook in a quiet area of the home, incorporating earthy colours, and placing meaningful symbols of wisdom, the individual experienced a transformative shift in their learning environment. The knowledge nook became a haven for concentrated study, contributing to an enhanced sense of intellectual fulfilment.

As we conclude our exploration of Chapter 10, the principles of Feng Shui unveil the profound impact of intentional design on the realms of creativity and knowledge within our living spaces. From activating the Knowledge gua to crafting mindful spaces in study areas, designated corners, and even outdoor environments, every adjustment contributes to the cultivation of positive energy that inspires innovation and intellectual growth.

Armed with the wisdom of Feng Shui, you now possess the tools to infuse your surroundings with the energy of creativity and knowledge. Whether it's the deliberate arrangement of your study space, the mindful selection of colours, or the incorporation of personalized symbols, each element plays a crucial role in creating an environment that stimulates the mind and unleashes your creative and intellectual potential.

In the forthcoming chapters, we will continue our exploration of Feng Shui, delving into advanced techniques, case studies, and practical applications that further illuminate the transformative power of this ancient practice. So, with the principles of creativity and knowledge as your guide, let the journey toward unlocking your mind's full potential continue, guided by the timeless wisdom of Feng Shui.

Chapter 11: Feng Shui for Personal Empowerment: Cultivating Inner Strength and Balance

In the intricate tapestry of Feng Shui, personal empowerment emerges as a central theme, weaving through the principles and practices of this ancient art. Chapter 11 embarks on a journey to explore the ways in which Feng Shui can be harnessed to cultivate inner strength, balance, and a profound sense of personal empowerment. By understanding the interplay of energy within our living spaces, incorporating auspicious symbols, and making intentional design choices, individuals can create environments that support and amplify their journey toward personal empowerment.

Foundations of Personal Empowerment in Feng Shui

Feng Shui views personal empowerment as a holistic endeavour, intertwining the physical, emotional, and spiritual aspects of an individual. The principles guiding personal empowerment in Feng Shui are rooted in creating environments that align with one's authentic self, fostering a sense of purpose, and providing a sanctuary for self-discovery.

The Bagua Map: Navigating the Path to Empowerment

As established in earlier chapters, the Bagua Map serves as a foundational tool in Feng Shui, guiding us to understand the specific areas of our homes associated with personal empowerment. The Personal Growth and Self-Cultivation gua, typically located in the centre of the Bagua, becomes the focal point for activating and enhancing the energy of empowerment.

Activating the Centre Gua:

To activate the Centre gua, focus on the central area of your home or individual rooms. Introduce elements, colours, and symbols associated with personal growth and self-cultivation to amplify the energy in this key zone. This may involve using earthy colours, incorporating symbols of balance, and placing items that evoke a sense of inner strength.

Earth Element for Grounding:

In Feng Shui, the Earth element symbolizes stability and grounding, foundational for personal empowerment. Introduce Earth elements in the central area through decor, such as stones, crystals, or earthy tones. These elements contribute to a grounded and balanced energy, supporting the journey toward personal empowerment.

Colours for Balance:

Colours play a pivotal role in Feng Shui, each associated with specific elements and energies. For areas related to personal empowerment, incorporating auspicious colours is key. Hues of yellow and earthy tones are particularly favourable. These colours not only activate the Centre gua but also resonate with the energy of balance, self-discovery, and empowerment.

Symbolic Representation of Empowerment:

Infuse the central area with symbols that represent personal empowerment and self-cultivation. Consider incorporating items such as meaningful artwork, sculptures, or symbols that resonate with your sense of purpose and inner strength. These symbolic elements serve as visual reminders of your journey toward personal empowerment.

The Power of Intention: Creating Empowering Environments

Feng Shui emphasizes the power of intention in shaping our environments. By aligning our living spaces with our intentions for personal empowerment, we harness the energy of our surroundings to support and amplify our inner strength.

Setting Clear Intentions:

Begin the journey toward personal empowerment by setting clear and positive intentions. Reflect on your goals, aspirations, and the qualities you wish to cultivate within yourself. Whether it's a sense of confidence, resilience, or balance, articulate your intentions with clarity and sincerity.

Mindful Arrangement of Spaces:

Arrange your living spaces in alignment with your intentions for personal empowerment. This may involve decluttering and organizing, creating designated areas that reflect your goals, and eliminating items that do not resonate with your sense of empowerment. Mindful arrangement promotes a harmonious flow of energy, supporting your journey toward inner strength.

Visual Representations of Empowerment:

Use visual representations that embody the qualities of personal empowerment. This could include artwork, quotes, or symbols that inspire and uplift. Surround yourself with images and objects that serve as constant reminders of your inner strength and the path toward empowerment.

Sacred Spaces for Self-Reflection:

Designate sacred spaces within your home for self-reflection and meditation. Create a tranquil corner or room where you can connect with your inner self. Incorporate elements such as cushions, candles, or spiritual symbols that enhance the energy of self-discovery and empowerment.

Balancing Yin and Yang Energies: The Essence of Empowerment

Feng Shui emphasizes the balance of Yin and Yang energies as a fundamental principle in cultivating personal empowerment. By harmonizing the receptive and active qualities within our living spaces, we create an environment that supports a balanced and empowered state of being.

Creating Yin Spaces for Reflection:

Designate Yin spaces within your home for moments of quiet reflection and contemplation. These spaces could include reading nooks, meditation corners, or areas with soft lighting and comfortable seating. Yin spaces promote a sense of introspection and inner balance, contributing to personal empowerment.

Infusing Yang Energies for Action:

Introduce Yang energies in areas where action and productivity are essential. This could be your workspace, exercise area, or any space where you engage in dynamic activities. Yang energies foster a sense of vitality, motivation, and empowerment, aligning with the active aspect of personal growth.

Balance in Colour Choices:

Choose a balance of colours that represent both Yin and Yang energies. Earthy tones, such as browns and yellows, contribute to a grounded and stable energy associated with Yin. Combining these with pops of vibrant colours, such as reds or oranges, infuses Yang energy, creating a harmonious balance that supports personal empowerment.

Flow of Energy Through Movement:

Ensure a smooth flow of energy through movement within your living spaces. Arrange furniture and create pathways that allow energy to circulate freely. Incorporate elements of movement, such as flowing curtains or mobiles, to promote a dynamic and empowered energy flow.

Personal Empowerment Altars: A Symbolic Journey Within

Creating a personal empowerment altar is a potent practice in Feng Shui, serving as a symbolic representation of your journey toward inner strength and balance.

Selecting Meaningful Objects:

Choose objects that hold personal significance and align with your intentions for empowerment. This could include crystals, affirmations, symbolic figurines, or items that evoke a sense of personal strength. Each object on the altar becomes a tangible representation of your empowered self.

Arranging with Intention:

Arrange the objects on the altar with mindful intention. Consider the placement of each item and the energy it contributes to the overall altar. Arrange objects in a way that resonates with your sense of balance and empowerment. The altar becomes a sacred space for daily reflection and connection with your inner strength.

Cleansing and Energizing Rituals:

Engage in regular rituals to cleanse and energize your personal empowerment altar. This could involve smudging with sage or Palo Santo, using crystals to absorb and release energy, or incorporating rituals that hold personal significance. Cleansing rituals contribute to maintaining a vibrant and empowered energy on the altar.

Daily Reflection and Affirmations:

Make it a practice to spend a few moments each day in front of your personal empowerment altar. Reflect on your intentions, express gratitude for your strengths, and affirm your journey toward empowerment. This daily ritual becomes a powerful anchor for aligning with your inner strength and maintaining a balanced state of being.

Case Studies: Transformative Empowerment Journeys

To illustrate the transformative power of Feng Shui in cultivating personal empowerment, let's explore two case studies where intentional adjustments were made to create environments aligned with inner strength:

Case Study 1: Balancing Yin and Yang for Personal Empowerment

Challenge: A professional facing burnout sought to create a home environment that supported both relaxation and productivity.

Solution: By applying Feng Shui principles, including the creation of Yin spaces for relaxation and Yang spaces for focused work, the individual experienced a transformative shift in their energy. The harmonious balance between Yin and Yang energies in their living spaces contributed to a sense of overall well-being and personal empowerment.

Case Study 2: Personal Empowerment Altar for Self-Discovery

Challenge: An individual on a journey of self-discovery and empowerment wanted to create a symbolic space within their home.

Solution: By crafting a personal empowerment altar with meaningful objects, affirmations, and cleansing rituals, the individual established a daily practice of reflection and connection. The personal empowerment altar became a focal point for cultivating inner strength, balance, and a sense of purpose.

As we conclude our exploration of Chapter 11, the principles of Feng Shui illuminate the profound impact of intentional design on the journey toward personal empowerment within our living spaces. From activating the Centre gua to creating empowering environments that balance Yin and Yang energies, every adjustment contributes to the cultivation of positive energy that supports inner strength and self-discovery.

Armed with the wisdom of Feng Shui, you now possess the tools to infuse your surroundings with the energy of personal empowerment. Whether it's the deliberate arrangement of spaces, the mindful selection of colours, or the creation of personal empowerment altars, each element plays a crucial role in creating an environment that aligns with your authentic self and empowers your journey.

In the forthcoming chapters, we will continue our exploration of Feng Shui, delving into advanced techniques, case studies, and practical applications that further illuminate the transformative power of this ancient practice. So, with the principles of personal empowerment as your guide, let the journey toward cultivating inner strength and balance continue, guided by the timeless wisdom of Feng Shui.

Chapter 12: The Art of Feng Shui Consultation: Nurturing Harmony in Living Spaces

In the intricate dance between energy, intention, and environment, the role of a Feng Shui consultant becomes paramount. Chapter 12 delves into the art of Feng Shui consultation, exploring the principles, methods, and nuances involved in guiding individuals toward creating harmonious living spaces. Through a deep understanding of energy flow, the Bagua Map, and personalized adjustments, a Feng Shui consultant becomes a catalyst for transformation, facilitating a journey toward balance, well-being, and positive energy in the homes and lives of their clients.

The Essence of Feng Shui Consultation

Feng Shui consultation is a personalized and dynamic process, rooted in the ancient wisdom of energy alignment. A consultant serves as a guide, interpreting the unique energy patterns of a space and offering tailored recommendations to optimize the flow of chi. The essence lies in understanding the client's goals, aspirations, and challenges, and collaboratively crafting adjustments that resonate with their individual needs.

Understanding the Client's Objectives

Initial Consultation:

The journey begins with an initial consultation where the Feng Shui consultant engages in a detailed conversation with the client. Understanding the client's objectives, challenges, and aspirations provides the foundation for the consultation process. This phase involves exploring the client's lifestyle, preferences, and the specific areas of their life they seek to enhance through Feng Shui.

Assessment of Current Energy Flow:

A Feng Shui consultant conducts an assessment of the client's living space, analysing the current energy flow and identifying areas that may benefit from adjustments. This involves studying the layout, furniture arrangement, and decor choices to gain insights into the energetic dynamics of the space.

Introduction to the Bagua Map: Mapping Personalized Energy Zones

The Bagua Map serves as a fundamental tool in Feng Shui consultation, offering a framework for understanding the energy distribution within a space. This ancient map is overlaid onto the floor plan of the home, dividing it into nine distinct energy zones, or guas. Each gua corresponds to specific aspects of life, such as wealth, relationships, and health.

Energy Alignment with Bagua Mapping:

The consultant guides the client in understanding the Bagua Map and its application to their living space. By aligning the Bagua with the floor plan, personalized energy zones are identified. This mapping serves as the basis for addressing specific life areas, ensuring that adjustments are tailored to the client's unique goals.

Prioritizing Areas of Focus:

Together with the client, the consultant prioritizes areas of focus based on the client's objectives and the energy distribution revealed by the Bagua Map. This collaborative approach ensures that adjustments align with the client's intentions, creating a customized roadmap for enhancing specific aspects of their life.

Intuitive Analysis and Adjustments: The Artistry of Feng Shui

Beyond the systematic application of the Bagua Map, the artistry of Feng Shui consultation involves intuitive analysis and personalized adjustments that resonate with the client's energy.

Intuitive Sensitivity to Energy:

A skilled Feng Shui consultant possesses intuitive sensitivity to energy patterns within a space. This involves tuning into the subtle vibrations and resonances that may not be immediately apparent. Through this intuitive analysis, the consultant gains deeper insights into the energetic imbalances and potential blockages in the client's environment.

Customized Adjustments:

The art of Feng Shui lies in crafting adjustments that are not only aligned with the Bagua Map but also resonate with the client's personal energy. This may involve rearranging furniture, introducing specific colours, incorporating elemental symbols, or suggesting personalized enhancements that reflect the client's aspirations. The goal is to create adjustments that feel authentic and transformative for the client.

Cultivating Balance: Yin and Yang Energies in Consultation

A key aspect of Feng Shui consultation involves harmonizing Yin and Yang energies within a space, fostering balance and well-being.

Assessing Yin and Yang Dynamics:

The consultant evaluates the balance of Yin and Yang energies in different areas of the home. This assessment considers factors such as lighting, colour schemes, and the arrangement of furniture. The goal is to create a harmonious blend of receptive and active energies that support the client's overall well-being.

Adjusting Yin and Yang Elements:

Recommendations may include adjustments to enhance Yin energies in spaces where relaxation and rejuvenation are essential. This could involve introducing softer lighting, comfortable furnishings, and calming colours. Conversely, areas requiring more active energy may benefit from brighter lighting, vibrant colours, and dynamic decor choices.

Case Studies: Illustrating Transformative Consultations

Let's explore two case studies to illustrate the transformative power of Feng Shui consultation in creating harmonious living spaces:

Case Study 1: Enhancing Career and Success

Client Objective: A professional seeking to enhance career prospects and success in their home office.

Consultation Approach: The consultant, after mapping the Bagua and understanding the client's objectives, recommended strategic adjustments. These included repositioning the desk for a clear view of the entrance, incorporating elements of the Water element for career enhancement, and introducing vibrant colours to stimulate creativity. The result was a harmonized home office that supported the client's career aspirations.

Case Study 2: Nurturing Family Harmony

Client Objective: A family desiring greater harmony and connection in shared spaces.

Consultation Approach: After mapping the Bagua and conducting a comprehensive assessment, the consultant prioritized adjustments in shared areas. Recommendations included rearranging furniture for better flow, incorporating Earth element decor for stability, and introducing symbols of unity. The family reported a noticeable improvement in the atmosphere, with increased communication and a sense of togetherness.

Empowering Clients: Education and Long-Term Impact

Feng Shui consultation goes beyond immediate adjustments; it empowers clients with knowledge and insights for long-term well-being.

Client Education:

A crucial aspect of Feng Shui consultation involves educating clients about the principles and practices. By imparting an understanding of energy flow, the Bagua Map, and the impact of intentional adjustments, clients are empowered to make informed decisions about their living spaces.

Implementing Sustainable Practices:

Consultants guide clients in implementing sustainable Feng Shui practices that align with their lifestyle. This may include ongoing adjustments, mindful decor choices, and periodic assessments to ensure the continuous flow of positive energy in their homes.

Ethical Considerations and Confidentiality

Feng Shui consultants adhere to ethical standards and prioritize client confidentiality throughout the consultation process.

Respecting Client Privacy:

Consultants recognize the personal nature of their work and prioritize client privacy. Information shared during consultations, including personal goals and challenges, is treated with the utmost confidentiality.

Transparent Communication:

Transparent communication is paramount in Feng Shui consultation. Consultants clearly explain the principles behind their recommendations, ensuring that clients have a comprehensive understanding of the adjustments proposed for their living spaces.

Conclusion: Facilitating Transformations with Feng Shui Consultation

As we conclude our exploration of Chapter 12, the art of Feng Shui consultation emerges as a transformative process, weaving together intuition, personalized adjustments, and a deep understanding of energy dynamics. From the initial client conversation and the mapping of the Bagua to the artistry of intuitive analysis and long-term empowerment, every step contributes to the harmonization of living spaces and the well-being of individuals and families.

Armed with the wisdom of Feng Shui consultation, practitioners possess the tools to guide others on a journey toward balance, harmony, and positive energy. In the forthcoming chapters, we will continue our exploration of advanced techniques, case studies, and practical applications that further illuminate the transformative power of this ancient practice. So, with the principles of Feng Shui consultation as your guide, let the journey toward creating harmonious living spaces for yourself and others continue, guided by the timeless wisdom of Feng Shui.

Chapter 13: Feng Shui in Architecture and Design: Building Harmonious Spaces

In the realm of architecture and design, Feng Shui emerges as a guiding principle, influencing the creation of spaces that resonate with positive energy and harmony. Chapter 13 delves into the integration of Feng Shui in architecture and design, exploring how the ancient principles of energy flow, balance, and intention can shape the physical structures we inhabit. From the layout of buildings to the selection of materials and the incorporation of symbolic elements, Feng Shui in architecture becomes a transformative force in creating environments that nurture well-being and connection.

The Fusion of Feng Shui and Architecture

Understanding Energy Flow in Architectural Design:

Feng Shui in architecture revolves around the mindful consideration of energy flow within and around buildings. Architects, drawing inspiration from this ancient practice, seek to create structures that facilitate the smooth circulation of chi, ensuring a harmonious balance of energy within the built environment. This involves strategic placement of entrances, windows, and internal spaces to optimize the flow of positive energy.

Site Selection and Orientation:

Fundamental to Feng Shui in architecture is the careful selection of building sites and the orientation of structures. The natural elements surrounding a site, such as mountains, water bodies, and vegetation, influence energy patterns. Architects align buildings with auspicious directions and consider the impact of natural features, harmonizing the structure with its surroundings.

Balancing Yin and Yang in Architectural Elements:

Architectural design embraces the balance of Yin and Yang energies, incorporating elements that evoke both receptivity and activity. This balance is reflected in the choice of materials, colours, and shapes. For instance, the use of curves and natural materials introduces Yin qualities, while angular shapes and vibrant colours contribute Yang energy. The interplay of these elements creates a dynamic and balanced architectural composition.

The Bagua Map as a Blueprint for Design

Translating Bagua Principles into Architecture:

Architects versed in Feng Shui use the Bagua Map as a blueprint for design, aligning the principles of energy distribution with the layout of buildings. Each gua of the Bagua corresponds to specific aspects of life, influencing design decisions to enhance corresponding areas within the structure. For instance, the Wealth gua may influence the design of financial institutions, encouraging the incorporation of elements associated with abundance and prosperity.

Personalized Design Solutions:

Feng Shui in architecture offers personalized design solutions based on the specific needs and goals of the occupants. Whether designing a residence, workplace, or public space, architects consider the Bagua principles to tailor the architectural elements, creating an environment that supports the well-being and aspirations of those who inhabit it.

Sacred Geometry and Feng Shui: The Alchemy of Design

Geometry as a Channel for Energy:

Feng Shui in architecture often integrates sacred geometry, viewing specific geometric shapes as channels for energy flow. Architects incorporate shapes such as circles, squares, and rectangles, each carrying unique energetic qualities. For example, a circular design may promote unity and balance, while squares and rectangles contribute a sense of stability and order.

Mandala and Architectural Design:

The ancient art of mandala creation finds expression in architectural design influenced by Feng Shui. Architects utilize mandala patterns and principles to organize spaces and elements within a structure. This intentional arrangement aligns with the circular and symmetrical qualities of mandalas, fostering a sense of unity and balance in architectural design.

Sustainable Architecture and Feng Shui: A Synergistic Approach

Natural Elements and Sustainability:

Feng Shui principles align seamlessly with the tenets of sustainable architecture. The emphasis on natural elements, such as wood, stone, and water, aligns with sustainable practices that prioritize eco-friendly materials. Architects committed to both Feng Shui and sustainability integrate green building practices, ensuring harmony not only in energy flow but also in environmental impact.

Energy-Efficient Design:

The concept of energy efficiency in modern architecture aligns with the principles of Feng Shui. Architects design buildings with optimal natural lighting, ventilation, and energy conservation. This approach not only enhances the well-being of occupants but also resonates with the Feng Shui emphasis on creating environments that are in harmony with natural elements.

Symbolic Elements in Architectural Design

Integrating Feng Shui Symbols:

Feng Shui in architecture often involves the incorporation of symbolic elements that carry positive energy. Architects strategically place symbols such as dragons, turtles, or auspicious plants in designs to enhance specific areas within a building. These symbols serve as visual anchors, infusing the space with intention and positive energy.

Water Features for Wealth and Abundance:

Water features, a prominent element in Feng Shui, find their way into architectural designs. Whether in the form of fountains, ponds, or reflective pools, water features are strategically placed to activate the Wealth gua. The reflective and flowing qualities of water symbolize abundance and prosperity, creating a harmonious energy within the space.

Case Studies: Architectural Transformations Through Feng Shui

Let's explore two case studies illustrating the transformative impact of Feng Shui in architectural design:

Case Study 1: A Feng Shui-Inspired Residence

Design Objective: A family sought a home that aligned with their values of balance and prosperity.

Architectural Approach: The architect applied Feng Shui principles, selecting a site with favourable energy flow, optimizing natural light, and incorporating elements symbolizing prosperity. The result was a residence that not only met the family's functional needs but also became a harmonious space supporting their well-being.

Case Study 2: Feng Shui-Influenced Workplace

Design Objective: A business owner aimed to create a workplace that fostered creativity and collaboration.

Architectural Approach: The architect, incorporating Feng Shui principles, designed collaborative spaces with natural light, introduced symbolic elements representing innovation, and aligned workstations with the Bagua Map. The workplace transformation resulted in increased employee satisfaction and a conducive environment for innovative thinking.

Education and Collaboration: Empowering Architects with Feng Shui Wisdom

Feng Shui Integration in Architectural Education:

The integration of Feng Shui principles in architectural education empowers future architects with a holistic understanding of design. Courses and workshops that explore the synergy between ancient wisdom and contemporary architectural practices enhance the skill set of aspiring architects, fostering a new generation that values both aesthetics and energy flow.

Collaboration Between Architects and Feng Shui Experts:

Collaboration between architects and Feng Shui experts enriches the design process. Architects, recognizing the value of Feng Shui principles, collaborate with experts to ensure a comprehensive approach to energy flow, symbolism, and intention. This synergy results in buildings that not only showcase architectural prowess but also resonate with positive energy.

Challenges and Considerations in Feng Shui Integration

Balancing Aesthetics and Functionality:

Architects face the challenge of balancing the aesthetic appeal of a design with its functionality when integrating Feng Shui principles. Striking the right equilibrium ensures that the architectural masterpiece not only looks appealing but also fosters positive energy and well-being.

Client Awareness and Acceptance:

Educating clients about the integration of Feng Shui in architectural design may present a challenge. Architects need effective communication skills to convey the benefits and rationale behind Feng Shui principles, ensuring client awareness and acceptance of the design approach.

As we conclude our exploration of Chapter 13, the fusion of Feng Shui and architecture emerges as a powerful synergy, shaping spaces that transcend mere physical structures. From the strategic alignment of buildings with natural elements to the integration of sacred geometry, symbolic elements, and sustainable practices, Feng Shui in architecture becomes a transformative force that nurtures well-being and connection.

Armed with the wisdom of Feng Shui integration, architects possess the tools to create spaces that not only captivate the eye but also resonate with positive energy. In the forthcoming chapters, we will continue our exploration of advanced techniques, case studies, and practical applications that further illuminate the transformative power of this ancient practice. So, with the principles of Feng Shui in architecture as your guide, let the journey toward building harmonious spaces continue, guided by the timeless wisdom of Feng Shui.

Chapter 14: Feng Shui Gardens and Landscaping: Cultivating Harmony in Outdoor Spaces

In the realm of Feng Shui, the principles of harmony, balance, and energy flow extend beyond the confines of buildings to embrace the outdoors. Chapter 14 explores the art of Feng Shui gardens and landscaping, unravelling the ways in which intentional design and alignment with natural elements create outdoor spaces that resonate with positive energy. From the layout of garden features to the selection of plants and the integration of symbolic elements, Feng Shui gardens become an extension of the ancient practice, fostering well-being and connection with nature.

The Essence of Feng Shui Gardens and Landscaping

Harmonizing with Nature:

Feng Shui gardens emphasize harmonizing outdoor spaces with the natural environment. Landscaping decisions take into account the flow of energy, the balance of elements, and the creation of a tranquil and balanced atmosphere. By aligning garden design with Feng Shui principles, individuals can cultivate outdoor spaces that not only enhance the beauty of their surroundings but also promote a sense of well-being.

Creating a Sanctuary for Chi:

In Feng Shui, chi represents the vital life force energy. Gardens and outdoor spaces are viewed as sanctuaries for chi, where the energy can circulate freely and nourish the surroundings. Through thoughtful landscaping, individuals can optimize the flow of chi, creating a garden that radiates positive energy and promotes a harmonious connection between nature and the inhabitants.

Key Elements of Feng Shui Gardens and Landscaping

Water Features for Flowing Energy:

Water is a central element in Feng Shui gardens, symbolizing abundance, and prosperity. Incorporating water features such as fountains, ponds, or streams enhances the flow of energy within the garden. Strategically placing water elements encourages positive chi, creating a sense of tranquility and balance.

Rock Arrangements for Stability:

Rocks and stones are employed to anchor and stabilize the energy in Feng Shui gardens. These elements symbolize the Earth element, contributing a sense of grounding and stability to the outdoor space. Thoughtful rock arrangements, whether in the form of pathways, sculptures, or rock gardens, foster a harmonious balance of energy.

Plant Selection and Symbolism:

The selection of plants in Feng Shui gardens goes beyond aesthetic considerations; it involves incorporating plants with symbolic significance. Different plants represent various elements and energies, contributing to the overall balance of the garden. For example, bamboo symbolizes flexibility and resilience, while cherry blossoms embody the fleeting beauty of life.

Garden Layout and the Bagua Map:

Feng Shui gardens often mirror the principles of the Bagua Map, with specific areas designated for different aspects of life. Aligning the garden layout with the Bagua allows individuals to enhance specific areas, such as wealth, health, or relationships, through intentional landscaping choices.

The Bagua Map as a Blueprint for Garden Design

Mapping Garden Zones:

Applying the Bagua Map to garden design involves mapping specific zones to corresponding areas of life. Each gua is associated with an element, colour, and aspect of life. By aligning garden features and plant selections with the Bagua, individuals can create an outdoor space that resonates with their intentions and enhances specific aspects of their lives.

Activating Gua Energies:

Feng Shui gardens leverage the Bagua Map to activate energies in different guas. For instance, introducing red flowers or decor in the Fame gua enhances recognition and reputation, while placing water features in the Wealth gua stimulates abundance. Garden design becomes a deliberate and symbolic expression of the individual's aspirations.

Intentional Planting and Design Strategies

Colour Harmony in Plant Selection:

Feng Shui gardens emphasize the harmonious interplay of colours, each associated with specific elements and energies. Thoughtful plant selection based on colour harmony contributes to the overall balance of the garden. For example, the Wood element is represented by green plants, while red or purple flowers embody the Fire element. A well-balanced colour palette enhances the visual appeal and energetic resonance of the garden.

Mindful Tree Placement:

Trees play a significant role in Feng Shui gardens, symbolizing longevity and strength. Mindful placement of trees involves considering factors such as size, shape, and the energy they bring to the space. Trees with lush, healthy foliage contribute vibrant Wood energy, while those with strong trunks and roots embody grounding Earth energy.

Flowing Paths and Walkways:

The layout of paths and walkways in Feng Shui gardens is designed to facilitate the smooth flow of energy. Curving paths with gentle turns create a meandering flow, preventing stagnant chi. Integrating pathways that guide individuals through different garden zones encourages a dynamic energy circulation, enhancing the overall experience of the outdoor space.

Symbolic Elements and Garden Features

Statues and Sculptures:

Statues and sculptures in Feng Shui gardens serve as symbolic elements, representing various aspects of life. For example, a turtle sculpture embodies stability and longevity, while a dragon symbolizes strength and protection. Thoughtfully placed sculptures become visual anchors, infusing the garden with intention and positive energy.

Zen Gardens for Tranquility:

Zen gardens, inspired by Japanese design principles, find resonance in Feng Shui. These minimalist and contemplative spaces incorporate elements such as sand, rocks, and carefully placed plants to create a sense of tranquility and mindfulness. Zen gardens serve as havens for reflection and meditation, fostering a serene and balanced atmosphere.

Case Studies: Transformative Feng Shui Gardens

Let's explore two case studies illustrating the transformative impact of Feng Shui in garden design:

Case Study 1: Enhancing Family Harmony

Design Objective: A family sought to create a garden that fostered harmony and connection.

Landscaping Approach: The landscape designer applied Feng Shui principles, mapping the garden according to the Bagua. Water features were introduced in the Wealth gua, and family-oriented spaces were enhanced in the Family gua. The transformed garden became a space for shared activities and relaxation, promoting a sense of unity.

Case Study 2: Cultivating Serenity in a Zen Garden

Design Objective: An individual aimed to create a Zen-inspired garden for meditation and contemplation.

Landscaping Approach: The garden designer integrated Feng Shui principles into the Zen garden, selecting plants with symbolic significance and arranging rocks to enhance energy flow. The result was a tranquil space that provided a sanctuary for reflection and mindfulness.

Educational Gardens and Community Spaces: Sharing Feng Shui Wisdom

Feng Shui Gardens in Educational Settings:

Integrating Feng Shui principles in educational gardens enriches the learning environment. Schools and universities can design outdoor spaces that inspire creativity, focus, and positive energy. Educational gardens serve as living laboratories where students can engage with nature while benefiting from the harmonizing effects of Feng Shui design.

Community Spaces for Connection:

Public parks and communal outdoor spaces can embrace Feng Shui principles to foster community well-being. Thoughtful landscaping and the incorporation of symbolic elements create environments that encourage social interaction, relaxation, and a sense of unity. Community gardens become shared sanctuaries, enhancing the overall quality of life for residents.

Challenges and Considerations in Feng Shui Garden Design

Climate and Plant Adaptation:

Designing Feng Shui gardens requires consideration of climate and plant adaptability. Selecting plants that thrive in the local climate ensures the long-term success of the garden. Additionally, understanding the energy dynamics specific to the region contributes to effective Feng Shui garden design.

Maintenance and Sustainability:

Maintaining a Feng Shui garden involves regular care and attention. Sustainable landscaping practices, such as water conservation and eco-friendly maintenance, contribute to the overall harmony of the garden. Balancing the aesthetic appeal with sustainable practices ensures that the garden remains a source of positive energy over time.

As we conclude our exploration of Chapter 14, Feng Shui gardens emerge as sacred spaces where nature, intention, and energy converge. From the symbolic elements and intentional plant selection to the harmonious layout based on the Bagua Map, the art of garden design becomes a transformative journey. Whether creating a family-oriented garden, a Zen-inspired retreat, or a community space, the principles of Feng Shui guide individuals in cultivating outdoor environments that resonate with positive energy and harmony.

Armed with the wisdom of Feng Shui garden design, individuals, landscape designers, and communities possess the tools to create outdoor sanctuaries that enhance well-being and connection with nature. In the forthcoming chapters, we will continue our exploration of advanced techniques, case studies, and practical applications that further illuminate the transformative power of this ancient practice. So, with the principles of Feng Shui gardens as your guide, let the journey toward cultivating harmonious outdoor spaces continue, guided by the timeless wisdom of Feng Shui.

Chapter 15: Feng Shui and Technology: Navigating the Digital Landscape with Harmony

In the era of rapid technological advancement, the integration of Feng Shui principles with technology becomes a fascinating exploration of balancing ancient wisdom with the digital landscape. Chapter 15 delves into the relationship between Feng Shui and technology, unveiling how conscious design choices and intentional practices can harmonize the energy flow within our digital spaces. From mindful placement of electronic devices to the impact of digital clutter, this chapter guides individuals in navigating the technological realm with a focus on balance, positive energy, and well-being.

The Digital Landscape and Energy Flow

Understanding Chi in Digital Spaces:

In Feng Shui, chi is the vital life force energy that circulates through all aspects of our environment. The digital landscape, characterized by electronic devices, networks, and virtual spaces, is not exempt from the principles of energy flow. Conscious consideration of how chi moves within digital spaces becomes essential for creating harmonious and energetically balanced environments.

The Impact of Electronic Devices:

Electronic devices, such as computers, smartphones, and tablets, emit electromagnetic fields (EMFs) that can influence the energy in a space. Feng Shui principles guide individuals in mindful placement of these devices to minimize potential disruptions to the natural flow of chi. Positioning devices in ways that align with energy pathways contributes to a balanced and supportive digital environment.

Mindful Workspace Design in the Digital Age

Optimizing Desk Layout:

Feng Shui principles extend to the design of digital workspaces, emphasizing the importance of desk layout for optimal energy flow. Placing the desk in the command position, where one has a clear view of the entrance and is supported by a solid wall, fosters a sense of security and control. This arrangement contributes to a positive and focused work environment in the digital realm.

Ergonomics and Well-Being:

Ergonomic considerations in digital workspace design align with the principles of comfort and well-being in Feng Shui. Choosing comfortable and supportive furniture, positioning the computer at eye level, and incorporating natural lighting contribute to a harmonious and health-supportive digital workspace. The goal is to create an environment that promotes productivity and balance.

Digital Clutter and Energetic Impact

Clearing Digital Clutter:

Just as physical clutter can disrupt energy flow in a space, digital clutter can have a similar impact on the virtual environment. Feng Shui encourages individuals to declutter digital spaces by organizing files, emails, and applications. Clearing digital clutter not only enhances efficiency but also contributes to a sense of mental clarity and focus.

The Impact of Background Images:

Background images on digital devices can influence the energy of the workspace. Feng Shui principles suggest choosing images that inspire positivity, balance, and focus. Whether it's a serene natural landscape or a motivational quote, the background image contributes to the overall energetic atmosphere of the digital space.

Harmonizing Digital Spaces with Elemental Balance

Integrating Elemental Energy:

Feng Shui recognizes the five elements—Wood, Fire, Earth, Metal, and Water—as fundamental forces that influence energy dynamics. Integrating elemental balance in digital spaces involves selecting colours, themes, and imagery that represent the desired elemental energies. For example, incorporating blue hues for a sense of calm or fiery reds for motivation can contribute to a harmonious digital environment.

Balancing Yin and Yang Energies:

The balance of Yin and Yang energies is a foundational principle in Feng Shui. In the digital realm, achieving this balance involves considering factors such as screen brightness, colour temperature, and the overall visual atmosphere. Adjusting these elements contributes to a comfortable and balanced digital experience that supports both relaxation and focus.

Digital Feng Shui Practices for Home and Office

Creating a Digital Command Centre:

Designating a specific area as a digital command centre aligns with Feng Shui principles. This centralized space for electronic devices fosters organization and intentionality. Implementing a digital command centre involves mindful placement of devices, cable management, and the incorporation of elements that symbolize focus and productivity.

Optimizing Wi-Fi and Connectivity:

Feng Shui encourages optimizing Wi-Fi and connectivity for smooth energy flow. Positioning routers strategically, minimizing electronic interference, and creating a dedicated space for connectivity contribute to a harmonious digital environment. Ensuring a reliable and efficient digital infrastructure aligns with the principles of balance and positive energy.

Case Studies: Balancing Technology with Feng Shui Wisdom

Let's explore two case studies illustrating the transformative impact of integrating Feng Shui principles with technology:

Case Study 1: Harmonizing a Home Office

Challenge: A remote worker experienced challenges in maintaining focus and productivity in a home office.

Feng Shui Approach: Applying Feng Shui principles, the individual reorganized the desk to align with the command position, cleared digital clutter, and introduced elements representing concentration and creativity. The harmonized home office resulted in improved focus and a more balanced work experience.

Case Study 2: Enhancing Virtual Meetings

Challenge: A team faced disruptions and fatigue during virtual meetings.

Feng Shui Approach: The team integrated Feng Shui principles by optimizing the virtual meeting space, considering background imagery, and addressing digital clutter. By creating a visually balanced and energetically supportive environment, virtual meetings became more engaging, contributing to improved communication and team dynamics.

Educational and Professional Spaces: Integrating Feng Shui with Technology

Feng Shui in Educational Technology:

Educational institutions can apply Feng Shui principles when integrating technology into learning spaces. Mindful design of digital classrooms, consideration of device placement, and attention to the overall energetic atmosphere contribute to a positive and conducive learning environment.

Technology in Professional Settings:

Companies can benefit from integrating Feng Shui principles in the design of digital workspaces. This includes optimizing office layouts, considering the energetic impact of technology, and creating digital environments that support employee well-being and productivity. The intentional use of technology aligns with the broader goal of fostering a positive organizational culture.

Challenges and Considerations in Digital Feng Shui

Adapting to Technological Changes:

The fast-paced nature of technological advancements presents a challenge in maintaining digital Feng Shui practices. Individuals and organizations need to adapt Feng Shui principles to evolving technologies, ensuring continued harmony in the digital landscape.

Balancing Connectivity and Digital Detox:

While optimizing digital connectivity is essential, it is equally important to balance it with periods of digital detox. Feng Shui encourages individuals to establish boundaries, take breaks from electronic devices, and create moments of intentional disconnection to maintain overall well-being.

As we conclude our exploration of Chapter 15, the integration of Feng Shui with technology offers a holistic approach to navigating the digital realm. From mindful workspace design to clearing digital clutter and harmonizing elemental energies, individuals can harness the wisdom of Feng Shui to create balanced and positive digital environments.

Armed with the principles of digital Feng Shui, individuals, educators, and professionals possess the tools to navigate the technological landscape with intention and harmony. In the forthcoming chapters, we will continue our exploration of advanced techniques, case studies, and practical applications that further illuminate the transformative power of this ancient practice. So, with the principles of Feng Shui and technology as your guide, let the journey toward a balanced and harmonious digital experience continue, guided by the timeless wisdom of Feng Shui.

Chapter 16: Feng Shui and Sustainable Living: Harmonizing with the Earth

In the quest for balanced and harmonious living, Chapter 16 explores the synergy between Feng Shui principles and sustainable practices. Rooted in the interconnectedness of all things, Feng Shui and sustainable living converge to create a blueprint for mindful consumption, eco-friendly design, and a harmonious relationship with the Earth. From energy-efficient homes to conscious consumer choices, this chapter guides individuals on a transformative journey towards sustainable living inspired by the wisdom of Feng Shui.

The Earth Element in Feng Shui and Sustainability

Honouring the Earth Element:

Feng Shui recognizes the Earth element as a grounding force that symbolizes stability, nourishment, and sustainability. In sustainable living, individuals can embrace the Earth element by making choices that minimize environmental impact, prioritize ethical practices, and foster a sense of interconnectedness with the natural world.

Sustainable Practices as an Extension of Feng Shui:

Sustainable living becomes an extension of Feng Shui principles, emphasizing the importance of living in harmony with nature. From the materials used in construction to daily lifestyle choices, individuals can weave sustainability into the fabric of their lives, aligning with the core principles of balance and positive energy.

Eco-Friendly Home Design and Feng Shui Integration

Natural Materials and Feng Shui Harmony:

Feng Shui encourages the use of natural materials that resonate with the Earth element. Sustainable home design embraces this principle by incorporating materials such as bamboo, reclaimed wood, and recycled metal. The intentional use of these materials not only aligns with eco-friendly practices but also contributes to a harmonious and energetically balanced living space.

Energy-Efficient Homes:

Energy efficiency is a key consideration in both Feng Shui and sustainable living. Designing homes that optimize natural light, utilize renewable energy sources, and prioritize energy conservation aligns with the principles of balance and positive energy. This integration contributes to a home environment that nurtures both well-being and environmental responsibility.

The Bagua Map as a Guide for Sustainable Living

Mapping Sustainable Practices:

The Bagua Map serves as a guide for incorporating sustainable practices into different areas of life. Each gua corresponds to specific aspects, such as health, wealth, and relationships. By aligning sustainable choices with the corresponding guas, individuals can create a holistic and environmentally conscious lifestyle.

Sustainable Landscaping and Outdoor Spaces:

Feng Shui extends beyond the walls of the home to include outdoor spaces. Sustainable landscaping practices involve water conservation, native plant selection, and mindful design choices that align with the principles of balance and harmony. A sustainable garden not only enhances the aesthetic appeal but also contributes to the overall positive energy of the property.

Conscious Consumer Choices and Feng Shui Wisdom

Mindful Material Selection:

Feng Shui encourages individuals to be mindful of the materials they bring into their living spaces. Sustainable living aligns with this principle by promoting the conscious selection of materials with minimal environmental impact. Choosing products made from recycled, upcycled, or eco-friendly materials contributes to a home environment that resonates with positive energy.

Decluttering for Sustainability:

The practice of decluttering in Feng Shui is mirrored in sustainable living through the promotion of a minimalist and intentional lifestyle. Conscious consumer choices involve avoiding unnecessary purchases, reducing waste, and repurposing items to extend their lifespan. The decluttering process not only creates a physically spacious environment but also aligns with the principles of simplicity and balance.

Holistic Wellness and Eco-Friendly Practices

Natural Healing and Sustainable Living:

Feng Shui views the home as a reflection of one's well-being, and sustainable living aligns with this holistic perspective. Integrating natural healing practices, such as aromatherapy, herbal remedies, and eco-friendly wellness products, enhances the well-being of individuals while fostering a sustainable and harmonious living environment.

Holistic Health and Environmental Harmony:

Sustainable living goes hand in hand with holistic health, emphasizing the interconnectedness of personal well-being and environmental health. Choosing organic and locally sourced foods, practicing eco-conscious fitness activities, and embracing holistic wellness practices contribute to an overall lifestyle that resonates with positive energy and environmental harmony.

Eco-Friendly Practices in Building and Renovation

Green Building Principles:

Feng Shui aligns with green building principles, emphasizing the importance of sustainable construction practices. Green building involves using energy-efficient materials, incorporating renewable energy sources, and designing spaces that optimize natural resources. This approach not only aligns with the principles of balance but also contributes to the long-term well-being of both individuals and the planet.

Renovation with Sustainability in Mind:

Feng Shui wisdom guides individuals in renovating their homes with sustainability as a central consideration. From choosing eco-friendly paints and finishes to optimizing natural ventilation and lighting, renovations can be approached in a way that enhances the energy flow of the space while minimizing environmental impact.

Case Studies: Transformative Sustainable Living Inspired by Feng Shui

Let's explore two case studies illustrating the transformative impact of integrating Feng Shui principles with sustainable living:

Case Study 1: Sustainable Home Renovation

Challenge: A family sought to renovate their home while embracing eco-friendly practices.

Approach: Integrating Feng Shui principles, the renovation focused on natural materials, energy-efficient design, and sustainable landscaping. The transformed home not only reflected positive energy flow but also contributed to the family's commitment to environmental sustainability.

Case Study 2: Eco-Conscious Lifestyle Transition

Challenge: An individual aimed to transition to a more eco-conscious lifestyle.

Approach: Drawing inspiration from the Bagua Map, the individual aligned sustainable practices with specific guas. This involved mindful consumer choices, energy-efficient home adjustments, and sustainable landscaping. The transition to an eco-conscious lifestyle not only enhanced personal well-being but also contributed to a harmonious living environment.

Educational Initiatives and Community Sustainability

Feng Shui and Sustainable Education:

Integrating Feng Shui principles into sustainable education initiatives enriches the understanding of holistic living. Schools and educational institutions can incorporate these principles into curricula, teaching students about the interconnectedness of personal well-being and environmental sustainability.

Community Gardens and Sustainable Living:

Community gardens, aligned with Feng Shui principles, become spaces for collective sustainable living. Individuals can come together to cultivate eco-friendly practices, share resources, and create outdoor environments that resonate with positive energy. Community initiatives contribute to the broader goal of fostering sustainability on a larger scale.

Challenges and Considerations in Sustainable Living with Feng Shui

Budgetary Considerations:

Sustainable living choices may sometimes involve an initial investment. Individuals need to consider budgetary constraints and explore cost-effective ways to integrate eco-friendly practices into their homes and lifestyles.

Educational Awareness:

Promoting sustainable living requires educational awareness. Individuals may need guidance on how to align Feng Shui principles with sustainable practices and the benefits of creating a harmonious living environment for both personal and planetary well-being.

As we conclude our exploration of Chapter 16, the integration of Feng Shui with sustainable living emerges as a transformative journey toward balance, well-being, and environmental harmony. From eco-friendly home design to conscious consumer choices, individuals can draw inspiration from ancient wisdom to create living spaces that resonate with positive energy while nurturing the Earth.

Armed with the principles of sustainable living and Feng Shui, individuals and communities possess the tools to embark on a holistic journey towards harmony. In the forthcoming chapters, we will continue our exploration of advanced techniques, case studies, and practical applications that further illuminate the transformative power of this ancient practice. So, with the principles of Feng Shui and sustainable living as your guide, let the journey towards a balanced and harmonious existence continue, guided by the timeless wisdom of Feng Shui.

Chapter 17: Feng Shui Rituals and Ceremonies: Sacred Practices for Energetic Harmony

In the rich tapestry of Feng Shui, rituals and ceremonies weave a profound connection between the tangible and the intangible, inviting individuals to engage with the energies that surround them. Chapter 17 explores the sacred realm of Feng Shui rituals and ceremonies, unravelling the transformative power of intentional practices that harmonize the flow of energy within living spaces. From space-clearing ceremonies to auspicious rituals, this chapter delves into the ancient wisdom that elevates Feng Shui beyond a physical arrangement to a spiritual and energetic journey.

The Essence of Feng Shui Rituals

Intentional Energetic Alignment:

Feng Shui rituals are rooted in the intentional alignment of energy within a space. By engaging in specific practices, individuals seek to clear stagnant energy, invite positive chi, and create an environment that supports well-being on both physical and spiritual levels. The essence of Feng Shui rituals lies in the conscious connection with the energies that permeate our surroundings.

Connecting with the Sacred:

Feng Shui rituals go beyond the mundane aspects of space arrangement, inviting individuals to connect with the sacred dimensions of their living spaces. Whether performed for a specific life event, a change in circumstances, or the turning of seasons, these rituals serve as bridges between the material and the spiritual, infusing spaces with intention, reverence, and positive energy.

Space-Clearing Ceremonies: Clearing Stagnant Energy

Smudging and Incense Cleansing:

Smudging, often using sage or other cleansing herbs, is a common practice in Feng Shui rituals. The ceremonial burning of herbs clears negative or stagnant energy, purifying the space. Similarly, the use of incense in Feng Shui ceremonies serves to cleanse and uplift the energy, creating a sacred and harmonious atmosphere.

Bell and Sound Clearing:

Sound has a profound impact on energy, and Feng Shui rituals often incorporate the use of bells or chimes. Ringing a bell or creating intentional sounds with specific frequencies helps disperse stagnant energy and invite fresh, positive chi. Sound clearing rituals are particularly effective in spaces with heavy or stuck energy.

Auspicious Feng Shui Rituals for Home Blessing

New Home Blessing Ceremony:

Moving into a new home is a significant life event, and Feng Shui offers rituals to bless and harmonize the space. This ceremony may involve creating an altar with auspicious symbols, offering blessings from different traditions, and setting intentions for abundance, harmony, and protection in the new dwelling.

Renovation and Space Activation:

Before or after renovations, Feng Shui rituals can be performed to activate the energy of the space. This may involve blessing the construction materials, setting intentions for the renovated space, and incorporating symbols or objects with positive energy to enhance the overall harmony of the environment.

The Bagua Map in Ritual Practices

Aligning Rituals with Bagua Areas:

The Bagua Map serves as a guide in Feng Shui rituals, allowing individuals to align specific practices with different areas of their living spaces. For example, a ritual aimed at enhancing prosperity may be performed in the Wealth gua, while a ceremony for fostering love and relationships may be conducted in the Love and Marriage gua.

Rituals for Each Bagua Aspect:

Each gua of the Bagua Map corresponds to specific aspects of life, elements, and colours. Feng Shui rituals can be tailored to address the unique energies of each gua. Whether focusing on career advancement, family harmony, or personal growth, aligning rituals with the Bagua amplifies their effectiveness and resonance.

Intention Setting and Affirmation Rituals

Creating Sacred Altars:

Altars play a central role in Feng Shui rituals, serving as focal points for intention setting and affirmation practices. Individuals can create altars that represent their aspirations, incorporating symbols, objects, and colours associated with their goals. Altars become energetic anchors, amplifying the intentions set during rituals.

Affirmation Practices:

Affirmations are powerful tools for shaping the energy of a space. Feng Shui rituals often involve the recitation of affirmations that align with specific intentions. Whether spoken aloud or written and placed in a designated area, affirmations contribute to the vibrational frequency of the space, fostering a positive and supportive environment.

Seasonal Feng Shui Rituals

Aligning with Nature's Cycles:

Feng Shui emphasizes the connection between the natural world and the energy within living spaces. Seasonal rituals acknowledge and align with the cycles of nature, inviting individuals to attune their living spaces to the changing energies of each season. From spring cleaning ceremonies to winter solstice rituals, these practices enhance the harmony between indoor and outdoor environments.

Celebrating Lunar New Year:

The Lunar New Year holds special significance in Feng Shui, marking a time of renewal and fresh energy. Rituals associated with the Lunar New Year may include space-cleansing ceremonies, the placement of auspicious symbols, and the setting of intentions for prosperity, health, and joy in the coming year.

Personal and Spiritual Growth Rituals

Feng Shui Vision Board Ritual:

Vision boards are popular tools for manifesting goals, and Feng Shui rituals can enhance their effectiveness. Individuals can create Feng Shui vision boards by aligning their goals with specific Bagua areas, incorporating symbolic images, and placing the vision board in an energetically supportive location to amplify the manifestation process.

Meditative Practices:

Feng Shui rituals often involve meditative practices that facilitate a deeper connection with the energy of the space. Guided visualizations, mindfulness meditation, or energy-clearing meditations align individuals with the spiritual dimensions of their living environments, fostering personal and spiritual growth.

Case Studies: Transformative Feng Shui Rituals

Let's explore two case studies illustrating the transformative impact of Feng Shui rituals:

Case Study 1: New Beginnings Ritual

Challenge: A family faced challenges in adjusting to a new home and wanted to create a harmonious atmosphere.

Ritual Approach: The Feng Shui consultant guided the family in a space-cleansing ceremony using sage, followed by a New Beginnings Ritual. This involved setting intentions for each Bagua area, creating a sacred altar, and incorporating symbols of growth and prosperity. The ritual not only cleared stagnant energy but also infused the home with positive vibrations, supporting the family's transition.

Case Study 2: Career Advancement Ceremony

Challenge: An individual sought to enhance career prospects and attract new opportunities.

Ritual Approach: The individual performed a Career Advancement Ceremony aligned with the Career gua of the Bagua Map. This involved creating a dedicated altar with symbols of success, reciting affirmations for career growth, and visualizing the desired outcomes. The ritual served as a focal point for intention setting and energetic alignment, contributing to a positive shift in career dynamics.

Educational and Community Ritual Practices

Feng Shui Workshops and Ritual Sessions:

Educational institutions and community centres can offer workshops and ritual sessions that teach individuals how to incorporate Feng Shui rituals into their lives. These sessions provide practical guidance on space-clearing techniques, intention setting, and the art of creating sacred altars.

Community Ceremonies for Collective Harmony:

Community-based Feng Shui rituals can contribute to collective harmony and positive energy. Whether performed during community events or seasonal celebrations, these rituals unite individuals in a shared intention to enhance the energetic well-being of their communal spaces.

Challenges and Considerations in Feng Shui Rituals

Cultural Sensitivity:

Feng Shui rituals may draw from diverse cultural and spiritual traditions. It is essential to approach these practices with cultural sensitivity, respecting the origins and significance of each ritual. Individuals and practitioners should be mindful of cultural diversity and adapt rituals in a way that honors and includes diverse perspectives.

Personalization and Intent:

Feng Shui rituals are most effective when personalized to align with an individual's intentions and goals. Consideration should be given to the specific energies present in the space, personal beliefs, and the unique circumstances of each individual. Intent plays a crucial role in the success of Feng Shui rituals.

As we conclude our exploration of Chapter 17, the world of Feng Shui rituals and ceremonies unfolds as a sacred realm where intention, energy, and spirit converge. From space-clearing ceremonies that dispel stagnant energy to auspicious rituals that bless new beginnings, these practices invite individuals to cultivate a deeper connection with the energetic essence of their living spaces.

Armed with the wisdom of Feng Shui rituals, individuals and communities possess the tools to infuse their surroundings with intention, positivity, and spiritual resonance. In the forthcoming chapters, we will continue our exploration of advanced techniques, case studies, and practical applications that further illuminate the transformative power of this ancient practice. So, with the sacred practices of Feng Shui rituals as your guide, let the journey toward nurturing the soul of living spaces continue, guided by the timeless wisdom of Feng Shui.

Chapter 18: Feng Shui and Mindfulness: Cultivating Presence in Living Spaces

In the intricate dance between the external environment and internal consciousness, Chapter 18 explores the profound intersection of Feng Shui and mindfulness. Rooted in ancient wisdom and contemporary practices, this chapter unravels the symbiotic relationship between mindful awareness and the energetic harmony of living spaces. From the principles of mindful space arrangement to the transformative impact on overall well-being, the integration of Feng Shui and mindfulness becomes a gateway to cultivating presence and balance in the daily tapestry of life.

The Essence of Mindfulness in Feng Shui

Present Moment Awareness:

At the core of mindfulness is the practice of being fully present in the moment. In the context of Feng Shui, this awareness extends to the energetic qualities of living spaces. Mindfulness invites individuals to observe, without judgment, the energy flow, arrangement, and ambiance of their surroundings, fostering a deeper connection with the present moment.

Conscious Interaction with Spaces:

Mindfulness in Feng Shui goes beyond surface-level observations; it involves a conscious interaction with living spaces. Individuals are encouraged to engage with their environments with intention, whether arranging furniture, decluttering, or selecting decor. This mindful approach heightens sensitivity to the energetic dynamics within spaces, aligning with the principles of balance and positive energy.

Mindful Space Arrangement: A Symphony of Presence

Conscious Furniture Placement:

Mindfulness in Feng Shui starts with the intentional placement of furniture. Rather than haphazard arrangements, individuals are encouraged to consider the flow of energy in a space. Mindful furniture placement aligns with the principles of the Bagua Map, creating harmony and supporting the desired energies in different areas of the home.

Decluttering as Mindful Practice:

Mindfulness permeates the practice of decluttering in Feng Shui. It involves more than the physical act of removing excess belongings; it's a conscious release of stagnant energy. Mindful decluttering invites individuals to assess the significance of each item, letting go of what no longer serves them, and creating a space that resonates with clarity and purpose.

Breath Awareness and Energetic Flow:

Aligning Breath with Movement:

Mindful breath awareness enhances the practice of arranging and interacting with living spaces. Whether placing objects, arranging decor, or engaging in space-clearing rituals, aligning breath with movement fosters a state of calm presence. The breath becomes a guide, syncing with the energetic flow within the space.

Breathing Life into Spaces:

Mindfulness invites individuals to infuse living spaces with conscious breath. This practice involves visualizing the breath as a gentle, revitalizing force that permeates the environment. By consciously breathing life into spaces, individuals contribute to an energetic atmosphere that supports well-being and balance.

Mindful Colour Selection and Energetic Resonance

Colour as Expression of Energy:

Mindful colour selection in Feng Shui involves understanding the energetic qualities of each colour and its impact on the atmosphere. Mindfulness invites individuals to choose colours that resonate with their intentions and preferences while aligning with the principles of the Bagua Map. This intentional approach contributes to a visually harmonious and energetically balanced environment.

Visual Mindfulness Practices:

Mindfulness extends to visual practices that enhance energetic awareness. This may include gazing meditation, where individuals mindfully observe specific objects or colours in their living spaces. Visual mindfulness practices contribute to a heightened sensitivity to the subtle energies present, fostering a deeper connection with the surroundings.

Mindful Soundscapes and Harmonic Resonance

Conscious Listening Practices:

Mindfulness in Feng Shui incorporates conscious listening practices. Individuals are encouraged to be attentive to the sounds within their living spaces, whether it's the hum of appliances, the rustle of leaves, or the ambient sounds of nature. Conscious listening fosters an awareness of the acoustic environment and its impact on energy flow.

Sound Alignment with Intention:

Mindful selection of sounds, such as music, chimes, or nature sounds, becomes a way to align the energetic atmosphere with intention. Mindful soundscapes contribute to a harmonious living environment, creating resonance with specific energies and supporting the desired atmosphere within the space.

Mindful Rituals for Energetic Well-Being

Morning and Evening Rituals:

Mindfulness in Feng Shui can be woven into daily rituals. Morning and evening rituals may involve setting intentions for the day or releasing accumulated stress and tension. Mindful practices, such as breathing exercises, gentle movements, or a brief space-clearing ceremony, establish a positive and intentional energetic tone for the day.

Mindful Movement Practices:

Mindful movement, such as Tai Chi or Qi Gong, aligns with the principles of Feng Shui by promoting the flow of chi within the body and the surrounding environment. These practices cultivate mindfulness through intentional, slow movements, fostering a deep connection with the present moment and the energy within and around the individual.

Mindful Connection with Nature: A Source of Renewal

Nature as a Mindful Retreat:

Mindfulness in Feng Shui emphasizes the importance of connecting with the natural world. Individuals are encouraged to create mindful outdoor spaces or bring elements of nature indoors. This practice serves as a mindful retreat, allowing individuals to recharge and attune to the rejuvenating energies of the Earth.

Mindful Gardening Practices:

Gardening becomes a mindful practice in Feng Shui, aligning with the principles of nature and the seasons. Individuals can cultivate a mindful connection with their gardens by observing the growth cycles, practicing mindful planting, and creating outdoor spaces that reflect harmony and balance.

Mindfulness and the Bagua Map: A Holistic Approach

Mindful Exploration of Bagua Areas:

Mindfulness deepens the exploration of each Bagua area, allowing individuals to attune to the specific energies associated with different aspects of life. Mindful practices, such as meditation or visualization, can be tailored to align with the intentions related to each gua, fostering a holistic and balanced approach to energetic well-being.

Mindful Adjustments for Energetic Balance:

As individuals mindfully assess the energy within each Bagua area, adjustments can be made with intention. Mindful placement of symbols, decor, or colour enhancements aligns with the specific energies associated with each gua, contributing to an overall sense of balance and well-being.

Mindfulness in Feng Shui Consultations

Client-Centred Mindfulness:

Feng Shui consultations benefit from a client-centred approach that integrates mindfulness. Practitioners can guide clients in cultivating present moment awareness, helping them connect with the energies of their living spaces. Mindfulness enhances the client's ability to articulate intentions, preferences, and goals, creating a more personalized and resonant Feng Shui experience.

Mindful Space Analysis:

Mindfulness informs the process of space analysis during Feng Shui consultations. Practitioners observe the subtle energies, listen to the client's needs, and guide them in mindful practices that support the harmonization of their living spaces. Mindful space analysis contributes to a holistic understanding of the client's environment and the energetic dynamics at play.

Case Studies: Transformative Mindfulness in Feng Shui

Let's explore two case studies illustrating the transformative impact of integrating mindfulness with Feng Shui:

Case Study 1: Mindful Home Office

Challenge: A professional working from home sought to create a harmonious and focused home office environment.

Mindful Approach: The Feng Shui consultant guided the individual in a mindful decluttering process, intentional furniture arrangement, and the incorporation of calming colours. Mindful breathing practices were introduced to enhance focus and clarity during work hours. The transformed home office became a mindful sanctuary, supporting productivity and well-being.

Case Study 2: Mindful Family Living

Challenge: A family sought to create a mindful and harmonious living environment for all family members.

Mindful Approach: Mindful rituals, including morning intention-setting and evening gratitude practices, were introduced to the family routine. Mindful furniture placement and the use of nature-inspired decor enhanced the energetic balance of different areas. The family embraced mindfulness in their daily interactions, fostering a sense of unity and well-being.

Educational Initiatives: Integrating Feng Shui and Mindfulness

Mindful Feng Shui Workshops:

Educational institutions and community centres can offer workshops that explore the integration of Feng Shui and mindfulness. These workshops provide practical guidance on mindful space arrangement, breath-awareness practices, and mindful rituals that enhance energetic well-being.

Mindfulness Retreats with Feng Shui Focus:

Retreats that combine mindfulness practices with Feng Shui principles offer participants an immersive experience. These retreats may include mindful movement sessions, guided space-clearing ceremonies, and explorations of mindful living practices aligned with Feng Shui wisdom.

Challenges and Considerations in Mindful Feng Shui Practices

Cultivating Consistent Mindfulness:

Consistent mindfulness practice requires dedication and intention. Individuals engaging in mindful Feng Shui practices may face challenges in maintaining a consistent level of mindfulness. Awareness of these challenges and the incorporation of gradual, sustainable practices can support individuals on their mindful journey.

Balancing Intuition and Mindfulness:

Mindfulness in Feng Shui encourages individuals to be present and intuitive in their interactions with spaces. Balancing intuition with mindfulness involves cultivating a deep connection with the energetic qualities of the environment while remaining anchored in present moment awareness. Striking this balance contributes to a more authentic and resonant Feng Shui practice.

As we conclude our exploration of Chapter 18, the integration of Feng Shui and mindfulness unfolds as a mindful symphony, where the harmonious dance between energy and presence comes to life. From mindful space arrangement to breath-aware practices, the art of cultivating mindfulness enriches the tapestry of living spaces with intention, balance, and vibrant energy.

Armed with the principles of mindfulness and Feng Shui, individuals and communities possess the tools to infuse their surroundings with a sense of presence, fostering holistic well-being. In the forthcoming chapters, we will continue our exploration of advanced techniques, case studies, and practical applications that further illuminate the transformative power of this ancient practice. So, with the mindful practices of Feng Shui as your guide, let the journey toward a symphony of energy and presence continue, guided by the timeless wisdom of Feng Shui.

Chapter 19: Feng Shui Myths and Misconceptions: Unravelling the Truths Behind the Legends

In the vast realm of Feng Shui, myths and misconceptions have woven a tapestry of intrigue and confusion. Chapter 19 aims to dispel the fog surrounding common beliefs and misunderstandings associated with Feng Shui, providing clarity on the authentic principles that guide this ancient practice. From the symbolism of mirrors to the misconceptions about specific Feng Shui cures, this chapter unravels the myths that may hinder a genuine understanding of the transformative power of Feng Shui.

Myth 1: Mirrors Double Your Problems

Truth: Mirrors in Feng Shui are powerful tools, and the myth that they double your problems is a misconception. While mirrors do reflect energy, they also have the ability to expand and circulate positive energy. Strategically placing mirrors can enhance natural light, create a sense of spaciousness, and redirect chi flow. It's essential to understand the purpose behind mirror placement and use them mindfully to optimize their positive effects.

Myth 2: Red Door Equals Good Feng Shui

Truth: While a red door is often associated with good Feng Shui, it's not a one-size-fits-all solution. The belief that painting your front door red automatically attracts positive energy oversimplifies Feng Shui principles. The key lies in selecting a colour that harmonizes with the overall energy of the home and aligns with the occupants' aspirations. Each individual's energy blueprint is unique, and the colour choice should be based on careful consideration of the specific energies present in the space.

Myth 3: Feng Shui Is Only About Arranging Furniture

Truth: While furniture arrangement is a significant aspect of Feng Shui, reducing it to merely rearranging furniture oversimplifies the depth of this ancient practice. Feng Shui encompasses a holistic approach to harmonizing energy within living spaces. It involves mindful decluttering, intentional colour selection, and the incorporation of symbols and elements that resonate with the occupants' goals. True Feng Shui is a multifaceted exploration of the energetic dynamics in both the external environment and the internal self.

Myth 4: Feng Shui Is a One-Time Fix

Truth: Feng Shui is a dynamic and ongoing practice rather than a one-time fix. Energy is constantly in flux, influenced by changes in the environment, seasons, and life circumstances. The belief that a single Feng Shui adjustment will permanently resolve all issues is a myth. Regular assessments and adjustments are necessary to align the living space with the evolving energies and the occupants' changing needs.

Myth 5: Feng Shui Is Strictly Superstitious

Truth: While Feng Shui is deeply rooted in ancient Chinese philosophy and symbolism, dismissing it as purely superstitious overlooks the practical and psychological benefits it can offer. Feng Shui principles often align with common-sense practices, such as optimizing natural light, maintaining a clutter-free environment, and promoting a harmonious flow of energy. Beyond superstition, Feng Shui offers a pragmatic approach to creating living spaces that support well-being and balance.

Myth 6: Feng Shui Is Only for Wealth and Prosperity

Truth: While wealth and prosperity are commonly associated with Feng Shui, its scope extends far beyond financial success. Feng Shui addresses various aspects of life, including health, relationships, career, and personal growth. The practice aims to create a harmonious environment that supports the holistic well-being of individuals. Focusing solely on wealth overlooks the transformative potential of Feng Shui in enhancing the overall quality of life.

Myth 7: Feng Shui Is a Quick Fix for Personal Issues

Truth: Feng Shui is not a quick fix for personal or life issues. While it can positively influence the energetic dynamics of a space, personal growth and development require a comprehensive approach. Individuals seeking profound transformation should complement Feng Shui practices with self-reflection, personal goal-setting, and, if needed, professional guidance. Feng Shui serves as a supportive tool rather than an instant remedy for complex life challenges.

Myth 8: Feng Shui Is a Religion

Truth: Feng Shui is not a religion; it is a traditional Chinese practice rooted in the principles of Taoism and Confucianism. While it incorporates spiritual and symbolic elements, it is not a belief system in itself. Feng Shui is accessible to individuals of various religious backgrounds, and its principles can be applied without subscribing to a specific spiritual tradition. It is a practical and cultural approach to harmonizing energy within living spaces.

Myth 9: Feng Shui Requires expensive Cures and Items

Truth: Feng Shui does not necessitate expensive cures or items for it to be effective. While certain symbols or elements may be recommended based on Feng Shui principles, the focus should be on intention and alignment with the occupants' goals. Affordable and meaningful adjustments, such as incorporating plants, mindful decluttering, or rearranging furniture, can have a significant impact on the energy of a space.

Myth 10: Feng Shui Is Strictly Cultural and Cannot Be Adapted

Truth: While Feng Shui has deep cultural roots in Chinese philosophy, it is not exclusive to Chinese culture. Its principles can be adapted and applied in various cultural contexts. Feng Shui acknowledges the interconnectedness of energy and the universal principles of balance and harmony. Adaptations can be made to align with different cultural aesthetics and preferences while maintaining the core principles of energy balance.

Myth 11: Feng Shui Is Only Relevant for Homes

Truth: Feng Shui is not limited to residential spaces; it is applicable to a wide range of environments, including offices, businesses, and public spaces. The principles of Feng Shui can be adapted to suit the unique needs and energy dynamics of different settings. Applying Feng Shui in workplaces, for example, can enhance productivity, creativity, and overall well-being among employees.

Myth 12: Feng Shui Practitioners Can Instantly Solve All Problems

Truth: While Feng Shui practitioners can provide valuable insights and guidance, it's a myth that they can instantly solve all problems. Feng Shui consultations involve a collaborative process where practitioners work with clients to understand their goals, assess the energy of the space, and suggest adjustments. Positive results often require time and ongoing engagement with Feng Shui principles.

Myth 13: Feng Shui Relies Solely on Compass Directions

Truth: While compass directions play a role in traditional Feng Shui (known as Classical Feng Shui), it is not the sole determinant of its effectiveness. Form School Feng Shui, which focuses on the visible features of the environment, and the Black Hat Sect Feng Shui, which uses the Bagua Map without compass directions, are examples of approaches that do not heavily rely on compass readings. The key is to choose a method that resonates with the individual's preferences and goals.

Myth 14: Feng Shui Is a New Age Trend

Truth: Feng Shui is not a new age trend; it has ancient roots dating back thousands of years. While it has gained popularity in Western cultures in recent decades, Feng Shui has been practiced in China for centuries. Its enduring relevance is a testament to the profound impact it has had on the lives and environments of countless individuals throughout history.

Myth 15: Feng Shui Is Only About External Changes

Truth: While external changes in the environment are part of Feng Shui, it also emphasizes internal shifts within individuals. Mindset, intention, and personal energy play crucial roles in the effectiveness of Feng Shui practices. True transformation occurs when external adjustments align with internal shifts, creating a harmonious interplay between the outer and inner realms.

As we conclude our exploration of Chapter 19, it becomes evident that Feng Shui is a practice deeply rooted in ancient wisdom, offering transformative insights when approached with understanding and intention. Dispelling myths and misconceptions allow individuals to embrace the authentic principles of Feng Shui, unlocking the potential for positive energy, balance, and well-being within living spaces.

Armed with a clear understanding of Feng Shui's truths, individuals and communities can navigate the rich landscape of this ancient practice, integrating its principles into their lives in a meaningful and empowering way. In the forthcoming chapters, we will continue our exploration of advanced techniques, case studies, and practical applications that further illuminate the transformative power of this timeless practice. So, with the truths of Feng Shui as your guide, let the journey toward harmonious living continue, guided by the wisdom that transcends myths and stands firm in the tapestry of ancient knowledge.

Chapter 20: The Future of Feng Shui: Navigating Harmonious Living in a Modern World

As we stand at the crossroads of tradition and modernity, Chapter 20 delves into the exciting frontier of the future of Feng Shui. In a world marked by rapid technological advancements, shifting cultural landscapes, and a growing awareness of the interconnectedness of all things, the ancient practice of Feng Shui continues to evolve. This chapter explores the trajectory of Feng Shui into the future, examining its relevance in contemporary society, the integration of technology, and the potential for global resonance in fostering harmonious living.

Feng Shui in the Digital Age: Navigating Virtual Spaces

Virtual Feng Shui Consultations:

As technology becomes an integral part of our lives, Feng Shui practitioners are exploring virtual consultations. Through video calls, practitioners can assess the energetic dynamics of spaces remotely, offering guidance on mindful space arrangement, symbol integration, and adjustments that align with clients' goals. Virtual consultations provide accessibility and convenience, opening new avenues for the global dissemination of Feng Shui wisdom.

Augmented Reality Applications:

Augmented reality (AR) applications offer exciting possibilities for experiencing Feng Shui principles in real-time. Individuals can use AR tools to visualize the energetic flow, optimal furniture arrangements, and colour choices within their living spaces. This immersive approach enhances the practical application of Feng Shui in a tech-savvy world, allowing users to interact with the energetic aspects of their environments.

Feng Shui and Sustainable Living: A Holistic Approach

Eco-Friendly Design and Feng Shui:

The future of Feng Shui intertwines with the global movement towards sustainable living. Integrating eco-friendly design principles with Feng Shui enhances the practice's holistic approach. By harmonizing with nature, individuals can create living spaces that not only support personal well-being but also contribute to the health of the planet. Sustainable architecture, energy-efficient practices, and green living align with the core principles of Feng Shui.

Feng Shui for Eco-Cities:

The future holds the potential for the incorporation of Feng Shui principles in urban planning and the design of eco-cities. By considering the energetic aspects of city layouts, public spaces, and architectural designs, urban environments can be crafted to enhance the well-being of their inhabitants. The integration of Feng Shui in urban planning contributes to sustainable, harmonious cities that prioritize the balance between human life and the natural world.

Cultural Adaptations and Global Resonance:

Feng Shui Across Cultures:

The future of Feng Shui envisions its continued adaptation across diverse cultural contexts. As the practice transcends its Chinese origins, it has the potential to become a global language of harmonious living. Individuals from various cultural backgrounds can integrate Feng Shui principles into their lives, recognizing the universality of energy balance and well-being.

Global Collaboration in Feng Shui:

With the interconnectedness of the modern world, the future of Feng Shui holds the promise of global collaboration. Practitioners from different corners of the globe can exchange insights, share cultural variations, and contribute to a collective understanding of Feng Shui's diverse applications. This collaborative approach enriches the practice, fostering a global community dedicated to the principles of balance and harmony.

Scientific Exploration of Feng Shui Principles:

Quantifying Energy Flow:

The future of Feng Shui may witness a deeper integration with scientific methodologies. Researchers and scientists may explore ways to quantify and measure the subtle energies that Feng Shui addresses. This scientific exploration can contribute to a broader understanding of the energetic dynamics within living spaces, validating the experiential wisdom of Feng Shui with empirical evidence.

Neuroarchitecture and Feng Shui:

The emerging field of neuroarchitecture, which studies the impact of the built environment on the brain, aligns with the principles of Feng Shui. The future holds the potential for collaborative research that explores the cognitive and neurological effects of Feng Shui practices. Understanding how specific arrangements, colours, and symbols influence cognitive processes contributes to a more comprehensive integration of Feng Shui in architectural and design disciplines.

Mindful Living and Feng Shui:

Mindfulness-Based Feng Shui Practices:

The future of Feng Shui embraces the growing emphasis on mindful living. Integrating mindfulness practices with Feng Shui principles amplifies the transformative potential of both approaches. Mindful decluttering, intentional space arrangement, and conscious engagement with the energies of the environment become integral components of a holistic and mindful lifestyle.

Mindful Technology Use in Feng Shui:

As technology continues to evolve, the future of Feng Shui incorporates mindful technology use. Mobile applications, smart home devices, and digital platforms offer tools for individuals to engage with Feng Shui principles in their daily lives. Mindful technology applications can provide reminders for intentional space adjustments, guided meditations, and personalized Feng Shui insights tailored to individual needs.

Educational Initiatives and the Next Generation:

Feng Shui Curriculum in Education:

The future holds the potential for the integration of Feng Shui into educational curricula. From elementary schools to universities, educational institutions may recognize the value of teaching students about mindful living, energy balance, and the interconnectedness of the built environment with personal well-being. This educational initiative fosters a generation with a deeper appreciation for the holistic principles of Feng Shui.

Online Feng Shui Courses and Workshops:

The accessibility of online platforms contributes to the democratization of Feng Shui knowledge. The future sees a proliferation of online courses, workshops, and resources that empower individuals to learn and apply Feng Shui principles. This widespread dissemination of wisdom supports a global community of informed practitioners, creating a ripple effect of positive energy and harmonious living.

Challenges and Considerations in the Future of Feng Shui:

Balancing Tradition and Innovation:

The future of Feng Shui requires a delicate balance between preserving traditional wisdom and embracing innovative approaches. While adapting to modern contexts, practitioners must honor the foundational principles that have guided Feng Shui for centuries. Striking this balance ensures the continued authenticity and relevance of the practice.

Cultural Sensitivity in Global Applications:

As Feng Shui expands globally, practitioners must navigate cultural sensitivity to ensure respectful and inclusive applications. Understanding and respecting the diverse cultural contexts in which Feng Shui is practiced contributes to its harmonious integration across the world.

As we conclude our exploration of Chapter 20, the future of Feng Shui emerges as a dynamic and expansive tapestry, interwoven with tradition, innovation, and the universal pursuit of harmonious living. The practice, rooted in ancient wisdom, continues to evolve, and adapt to the complexities of the modern world. From virtual consultations to sustainable urban planning, Feng Shui navigates new frontiers while remaining anchored in its foundational principles.

Armed with the insights of the future, individuals and communities can embark on a journey of mindful living, co-creating spaces that resonate with balance, positive energy, and a deep connection to the world around them. The evolving landscape of Feng Shui invites us to embrace the infinite possibilities that lie ahead, ensuring that the timeless wisdom of this ancient practice continues to illuminate the path to harmonious living for generations to come.

www.ingramcontent.com/pod-product-compliance
Lightning Source LLC
Chambersburg PA
CBHW050819260726
48660CB00004B/1511